FIGHT CANCER
with
VITAMINS
and
SUPPLEMENTS

FIGHT CANCER

with

VITAMINS

and

SUPPLEMENTS

A GUIDE TO
PREVENTION AND TREATMENT

Kedar N. Prasad, Ph.D.
and
K. Che Prasad, M.S., M.D.

Healing Arts Press
Rochester Vermont

Healing Arts Press
One Park Street
Rochester, Vermont 05767
www.InnerTraditions.com

Healing Arts Press is a division of Inner Traditions International

Note to reader: This book is intended as an informational guide. The remedies,
approaches, and techniques described herein are meant to supplement, and not to be a
substitute for, professional medical care or treatment. They should not be used to treat
a serious ailment without prior consultation with a qualified health care professional.

Library of Congress Cataloging-in-Publication Data

Prasad, Kedar N.
    Fight cancer with vitamins and supplements : a guide to prevention and
treatment / Kedar N. Prasad and K. Che Prasad.
        p. cm.
    Rev. ed. of: Vitamins in cancer prevention and treatment. 1989.
    Includes bibliographical references and index.
    ISBN 0-89281-949-9
    1. Cancer—Diet therapy. 2. Vitamin therapy. 3. Dietary supplements.
4. Cancer—Chemoprevention. I. Prasad, Che. II. Prasad, Kedar N.
Vitamins in cancer prevention and treatment.

RC271.V58 P73 2001
616.99'40654—dc21

                                                        2001016762

Printed and bound in the United States

10 9 8 7 6 5 4 3 2 1

Text design and layout by Rachel Goldenberg
This book was typeset in Adobe Garamond with Frutiger as the display typeface

*This book is dedicated to Judy,
devoted wife and loving mother.*

Contents

Foreword

The public has become increasingly interested in personal health and has been besieged with recommendations from many different organizations and people. A particularly controversial area has been that of vitamins and cancer. Drs. Kedar Prasad and Che Prasad have prepared a useful and well-organized antidote to the mass of irresponsible information about vitamins. They open with a short, clever review of what is fact and what is fiction about micronutrients and cancer; this perspective alone is worth the purchase of this book.

The authors then present the potential role of micronutrients in the prevention and treatment of human cancers. Their review of laboratory and epidemiological evidence for certain micronutrients as natural inhibitors of cancer is clear and understandable to the average person. Their interim guidelines for micronutrient usage, diet changes, and lifestyle considerations for the prevention of human cancer are considered and reasonable. The distinction between the doses of nutrients that may be necessary for adequate nutrition versus cancer prevention is an important issue, one that they address from a balanced perspective.

Major new areas of research on the possible role of micronutrients in the treatment of cancer or in the alleviation of the effects of treatment for cancer are discussed. The authors give an overview of this rapidly developing field and view research results with cautious optimism. The list of more than one hundred internationally recognized clinical and laboratory investigators working in the area of vitamins, nutrition, and cancer is extremely valuable and one that we hope will be used by the public. As a physician who frequently sees bad results from the misuse of vitamins for nutrition or prevention or treatment of human cancers, I applaud Drs. Kedar Prasad and Che Prasad for their responsible presentation.

Frank L. Meyskens Jr., M.D.

Director, Chao Family Comprehensive Cancer Center,
University of California, Irvine

Preface

An increasing number of people interested in maintaining and improving their health are using supplementary nutrition to help achieve their goals. Recent studies estimate that more than 40 percent of people in the United States take some form of supplementary nutrition every day. Most of them are unaware of recent developments concerning nutrition and cancer, and many may be taking nutrients without reference to up-to-date scientific guidelines. It is well known that excessive consumption of certain nutrients can cause irreversible damage to the body. The consumption of the appropriate types and amounts of antioxidants, B vitamins, and minerals is essential for optimal health.

This book has two major purposes: to make the public, physicians, and health professionals aware of the results of recent research on the role of antioxidants, diet, and lifestyle in cancer prevention and as an adjunct to standard therapy in cancer treatment and to provide guidelines to develop individual dietary and supplemental nutritional programs for cancer prevention and treatment. Such programs must be developed in close consultation with physicians or other health professionals who are knowledgeable about nutrition and cancer. The cancer prevention program may be equally effective for maintaining good health and thus can prevent other chronic diseases, such as heart disease. We also have included a list of major scientific publications on micronutrients and cancer and a list of more than one hundred major international institutions where micronutrients are being studied in the prevention and treatment of cancer.

We would like to thank Charlotte Jensen for her editorial skills, and we offer a special thanks to Kathleen Prasad for her support.

Kedar N. Prasad, Ph.D.
K. Che Prasad, M.S., M.D.

1 Fact and Fiction about Antioxidants, Diet, and Cancer

Antioxidants are micronutrients that protect our bodies against damage caused by free radicals. Some antioxidants are made in the human body, and others are found in the diet. They are absolutely essential for our growth and survival. Free radicals are atoms or molecules with reactive oxygen that are formed as by-products whenever oxygen is used by cells. Free radicals can damage all parts of the cell, including the genetic material.

In recent years, many popular magazines and books have described new advances in research into the role of antioxidants and diet in cancer prevention and treatment. Unfortunately, many of these reports have produced contradictory claims regarding the usefulness of antioxidants for maintaining good health and preventing and treating cancer. As a result, a number of misconceptions concerning the value of supplementary micronutrients exist among the general public and most health professionals. Some of them are discussed herein.

1. **Fiction:** The more supplementary micronutrients, including antioxidants, you take, the better you will feel.

   Fact: This belief can be dangerous. Consumption of excessive quantities of certain micronutrients may cause severe damage. For instance, taking large amounts of vitamin A (50,000 international units [IU] or more per day over a long period of time) may lead to liver and skin toxicity. Vitamin A at doses of 10,000 IU or more can increase the risk of birth defects in pregnant women. Excessive intake of selenium (500 micrograms [mcg] or more per day over a long period of time) may cause cataracts (an eye disease in which the lens becomes opaque). Taking B_6 vitamins (50 milligrams [mg]/day or more over an extended period) can induce peripheral neuropathy (numbness in the extremities), which is reversible upon discontinuation of the vitamin.

2. **Fiction:** All the different forms of vitamins A, C, and E have similar effects on cancer cells.

   Fact: This statement has been proved untrue in many experiments. For example, retinoic acid, a product of vitamin A, and its derivatives are more effective than other forms of vitamin A, such as retinol, retinyl acetate, or retinyl palmitate, in reducing the growth of cancer cells. Vitamin E in the form of d-α-tocopheryl succinate is more potent than other forms, such as d-α-tocopherol, d-α-tocopheryl acetate, or d-α-tocopheryl nicotinate, in curtailing the growth of cancer cells. Vitamin C is sold commercially as ascorbic acid, sodium ascorbate, or calcium ascorbate. Ascorbic acid at high doses can cause upset stomach in some persons. Sodium ascorbate at high doses can increase the concentration of sodium in the urine, which has been shown to magnify the risk of chemically induced bladder cancer in animals. Calcium ascorbate appears to be the most suitable form of vitamin C.

3. **Fiction:** The addition of trace minerals, such as iron, copper, and manganese, to many antioxidant preparations containing vitamin C is good for your health.

   Fact: It is well established that vitamin C in combination with iron, copper, or manganese generates free radicals that can damage cells. In addition, the absorption of these minerals in the presence of antioxidants is enhanced markedly in the intestinal tract, which can then increase the body's storage of these minerals. Heightened iron storage in the body has been associated with many chronic diseases, such as heart disease, cancer, and neurological diseases.

4. **Fiction:** Frozen fruit juices and powdered drinks maintain the stated levels of vitamin C when stored in the refrigerator.

   Fact: Frozen fruit juices and powdered drinks may provide beneficial amounts of vitamin C when drunk immediately after preparation. When they are stored in a cold place and exposed to light and/or oxygen, however, the vitamin C in the solution rapidly deteriorates. After 24 hours, more than 50 percent of the vitamin C activity is lost. Orange juice in cartons may have more vitamin C than the orange juice in plastic containers, but repeated opening and closing diminishes vitamin C levels.

5. **Fiction:** Some people believe that to maintain good health or prevent cancer, they should take all their micronutrients once a day; others believe that taking micronutrients, such as vitamin C, once in a while (for example, only during a cold) is enough.

   Fact: The frequency with which one should take micronutrients depends upon the rate of degradation in the body. The biological half-life (the time it takes for the concentration of a vitamin in the blood to be reduced by 50 percent) of most antioxidants is about 6 to 12 hours. Ingesting micronutrients once a day cannot maintain constant levels of antioxidants in the blood. Taking micronutrients containing antioxidants orally twice a day (morning and evening), however, will achieve a more constant level of these nutrients in the body. Consuming antioxidants before a meal has the beneficial effect of reducing the formation of toxic chemicals during the digestion of food. Taking supplementary micronutrients once in a while has no real health value.

6. **Fiction:** Avoiding excessive red meat consumption has no role in preventing cancer.

   Fact: Excessive consumption of red meat in Western countries has been linked to the development of colon cancer, a finding that is supported by the fact that the incidence of colon cancer among Seventh Day Adventists, a religious group whose members are vegetarians, is extremely low. Heme, a component of hemoglobin in the red blood cell, is present in red meat and can cause increased proliferation of colon epithelial cells, which can contribute to the risk of cancer. For this reason excessive ingestion of red meat should be avoided.

7. **Fiction:** Supplementary micronutrients are not necessary for cancer prevention.

   Fact: There have been some flawed and poorly controlled intervention trials on supplementary antioxidants that suggest that they may not be helpful in cancer prevention. On the other hand, there are many well-designed animal studies, cell-culture studies, and a few human studies that indicate that many supplementary micronutrients are essential in lowering the risk of cancer.

8. **Fiction:** A balanced diet is sufficient for optimal protection against cancer.

Fact: The concept of a "balanced diet" is very general. A balanced diet alone may not be adequate for optimal protection against cancer. Trying to obtain the optimal levels of antioxidants, such as vitamins A, C, and E and β-carotene, at the appropriate times through a balanced diet only may not be possible or practical. In addition, all foods that we consume on a daily basis contain both protective and toxic substances. In order to maximize the intake of protective substances, supplementary micronutrients are important. For these reasons, supplementary micronutrients together with a healthy diet and lifestyle are essential for maximum protection against cancer.

9. **Fiction:** Our environment, including food and water, are already polluted, and we have to accept the increasing risk of cancer as a part of living in today's world.

    Fact: Although it is impossible to remove all cancer-causing substances from our environment, diet, and water, we certainly can lessen their cancer-causing actions with proper supplementary micronutrients and a healthy diet and lifestyle.

10. **Fiction:** Large amounts of zinc are necessary for maximal health and cancer prevention.

    Fact: Zinc is essential for our survival. It acts as a cofactor in many important biological reactions. Excess zinc, however, may block the absorption of selenium, an important anti-cancer agent, and may impair the function of mitochondria.

11. **Fiction:** Cancer is a disease of old people, so you don't have to worry as much about a child's nutrition with regard to cancer prevention.

    Fact: Although this may be true for some cancers (such as colon and prostate cancer), many cancers can develop at any age. Thus, cancer prevention through micronutrient supplementation and changes in diet and lifestyle is equally important for children.

12. **Fiction:** Most supplementary micronutrients, including antioxidants, pass out of the body in the urine and feces, so why take them?

    Fact: The absorption from the intestine of most orally ingested antioxidants is about 10 percent. Consumption of high doses of antioxidants can lead to increased levels of these nutrients and their products in the urine and feces. The presence of certain antioxidants in the intestinal tract may be beneficial, however, even if they are not totally absorbed into the bloodstream. Increased amounts of vitamin C and vitamin E (α-tocopherol) are needed in the stomach to lower levels of nitrosamine, a potent cancer-causing agent that is formed from nitrite-containing foods, such as bacon, sausage, hot dogs, or cured meat. In addition, these antioxidants can reduce the levels of toxins (mutagens) formed during digestion in the intestinal tract. For these reasons, higher than normal amounts of antioxidants in the feces and urine should not be considered wasteful, since they may have a beneficial effect in the body even without being completely absorbed.

13. **Fiction:** Supplementary vitamin C causes kidney stones.

    Fact: This effect has not been observed in normal adults. If the urine becomes acidic, some of the waste products in the kidney may solidify and form stones, but this biological phenomenon usually occurs if there is an imbalance in body chemistry such that acidic solutions cannot be neutralized in the blood. The body normally neutralizes any acidic solution that it takes in. In certain specific disease conditions in which one's body has lost this capacity, one should not take vitamin

C in large amounts. The link between vitamin C intake and kidney stones is derived from two observations: (1) persons taking vitamin C at high doses sometimes show increased excretion of oxalic acid in the urine, and (2) many persons who have kidney stones also have higher than normal levels of oxalic acid in the urine. These two separate observations have been interpreted to mean that high doses of vitamin C can heighten the risk of kidney stones. These observations may be unrelated, since there are no published data to support the conclusion that high doses of vitamin C produce kidney stones in healthy people.

14. **Fiction:** Supplementary antioxidants are addictive.

    Fact: Supplementary antioxidants are not addictive. People who are taking high doses of supplementary antioxidants should not stop abruptly, however, because the body's systems may have adjusted to higher doses of vitamins and sudden withdrawal may lead to symptoms of vitamin deficiency.

15. **Fiction:** Micronutrients alone are sufficient to treat all cancers.

    Fact: Because of the complexities of cancer, no antioxidants, individually or in combination, are sufficient to treat advanced cancer. Several micronutrients at high doses and in combination with standard therapy, such as radiation and chemotherapy, may be useful in the treatment of cancer. They also may help delay or prevent the recurrence of cancer. Using micronutrients in the treatment of cancer must be done according to a scientific rationale; otherwise they may be ineffective or even harmful.

16. **Fiction:** Beta-carotene acts only as a parent of vitamin A and has no function of its own.

    Fact: In addition to acting as a parent of vitamin A (one molecule of β-carotene produces two molecules of vitamin A), β-carotene has some biological effects that vitamin A does not. For example, β-carotene enhances the expression of the connexin gene, which produces a gap junction protein in cancer cells, but vitamin A has no such effect. A gap junction protein is important in holding two normal cells together. Amounts of this protein are decreased in cancer cells. Induction of this protein suggests that cancer cells can become more like normal cells. Vitamin A causes differentiation (a process of converting cancer cells to normal cells) in some cancer cells, whereas β-carotene does not have this effect. This complementary effect of β-carotene and vitamin A often is ignored. In fact, supplements of both β-carotene and vitamin A are essential for cancer prevention.

17. **Fiction:** All fat-soluble antioxidants are toxic to humans.

    Fact: Only vitamin A and vitamin D, when taken at high doses over a long period of time or during pregnancy, have been shown to be potentially toxic.

18. **Fiction:** Natural and synthetic antioxidants have similar effects on cancer.

    Fact: Natural vitamin E is more effective than synthetic vitamin E as an antioxidant and for other cellular functions. Natural β-carotene can limit the formation of radiation-induced cancer cells, whereas synthetic β-carotene cannot.

19. **Fiction:** High-dose antioxidants have similar effects on normal and cancer cells.

    Fact: High-dose antioxidants have been shown to inhibit the growth of cancer cells but have no such effect on normal cells.

20. **Fiction:** All antioxidants act on cancer cells in only one way. They destroy free radicals.

Fact: In addition to destroying free radicals, antioxidants have some biological effects on cancer cells that are independent of antioxidation, such as gene regulation and induction of differentiation in cancer cells.

21. **Fiction:** High-dose antioxidants alone or in combination protect cancer cells against damage caused by irradiation and chemotherapeutic agents.

    Fact: High-dose antioxidants, such as vitamin A, C, and E and β-carotene alone or in combination, can enhance the effect of irradiation and chemotherapeutic agents on cancer cells but not on normal cells. Other antioxidants, such as sulfhydryl (SH) compounds (glutathione), protect both cancer cells and normal cells against damage by irradiation.

22. **Fiction:** If you take supplementary micronutrients, you do not have to worry about a balanced diet or modification in lifestyle.

    Fact: Supplementary micronutrients and a healthy diet (low fat and high fiber) and lifestyle are equally important for optimal health and disease prevention.

Concluding Remarks

Many misconceptions exist regarding the value of specific micronutrients (including antioxidants) in health and in disease prevention and treatment. A few have been discussed in this chapter. Putting these myths to rest is a challenge for researchers, physicians, and other health professionals. Success in improving the health of the general population depends upon the success of educating people about these misconceptions. At this time, a few clinical trials studying the role of one or more micronutrients in cancer prevention are in progress. A small number of clinical studies assessing the role of several high-dose micronutrients, including antioxidants, in combination with standard therapy in cancer treatment are also under way, while others, including both pediatric and adult cancer patients, are in the planning stages. We recommend that you develop a guideline for micronutrient supplementation and modifications in diet and lifestyle for optimal health and for cancer prevention and treatment (see chapters 5 and 6) using this book in conjunction with consultation with your doctors and health professionals.

2 Free Radicals and Antioxidants

In the beginning, the earth's atmosphere had no oxygen. Anaerobic organisms, which can live without oxygen, thrived. About 2.5 billion years ago blue-green algae in the ocean acquired the ability to split water (H_2O) into hydrogen (H) and oxygen (O_2). This chemical reaction initiated the release of oxygen into the atmosphere. The increased levels of atmospheric oxygen led to the extinction of many anaerobic organisms, owing to oxygen's toxicity. This important biological event also led to the evolution of multicellular organisms, including humans, who utilize oxygen for survival.

Today the amount of oxygen in dry air is about 21 percent, and in water it is about 34 percent. To understand the role of free radicals and antioxidants in the human body, it is important to grasp the relationship between oxidation and reduction processes, which are constantly taking place in the body.

Oxidation and Reduction

Oxidation is a process in which an atom or molecule gains oxygen, loses hydrogen, or loses an electron. For example, carbon gains oxygen during oxidation and becomes carbon dioxide. A superoxide radical loses an electron during oxidation and becomes oxygen. Thus, an oxidizing agent is a molecule or atom that changes another chemical by adding oxygen to it or by removing an electron or hydrogen from it. Examples of oxidizing agents or processes are free radicals, ozone, and irradiation.

Reduction is a process in which an atom or molecule loses oxygen, gains hydrogen, or gains an electron. For example, carbon dioxide loses oxygen and becomes carbon monoxide, carbon gains hydrogen and becomes methane, and oxygen gains an electron and becomes a superoxide anion. Thus, a reducing agent is a molecule or atom that changes another chemical by removing oxygen from it or by adding hydrogen or an electron to it. All antioxidants can be considered reducing agents.

Free Radicals

Free radicals are atoms or molecules with unpaired electrons (reactive oxygen or reactive nitrogen) that are highly damaging. Most free radicals are very short-lived (10^{-10} seconds). They can damage DNA (deoxyribonucleic acid), RNA (ribonucleic acid), protein, membranes, fat, and other cell components. Free radicals commonly mediate the actions of a diverse group of toxins that can enhance the incidence of many human chronic diseases, including cancer.

Sources and Types of Free Radicals

Free radicals are derived from either oxygen or nitrogen. Most free radicals derived from oxygen are called *reactive oxygen species,* and those derived from nitrogen are called *reactive nitrogen species.* Examples of the former include superoxide anion, hydroxy radical, hydroperoxy radical, organic radical, peroxy radical, and hydrogen peroxide. Examples of the latter include nitric oxide, nitric dioxide, and peroxynitrite. Thus, the human body is exposed to several types of free radicals.

Processes That Generate Free Radicals

Free radicals are created during the intake of oxygen, in the course of infection, and during the oxidative metabolism of certain compounds. Mitochondria are elongated membranous structures in the cells that are responsible for producing energy. While generating energy, mitochondria utilize oxygen and produce superoxide anions, hydroxy radicals, and hydrogen peroxide as by-products. About 2 percent of the unused oxygen leaks out of mitochondria and makes about twenty billion molecules of superoxide anions and hydrogen peroxide per cell per day. During bacterial or viral infection, phagocytic cells (which destroy bacteria- or virus-infected cells) generate high levels of nitric oxide, superoxide anions, and hydrogen peroxide in order to kill infectious agents; however, they also can cause damage to normal cells. In the course of the metabolism of fatty acids and other molecules in the body, free radicals also are produced. Certain factors and agents, such as smoking, free iron, copper, and manganese, can increase the rate of production of free radicals. Thus, the human body is exposed constantly to varying levels of free radicals. Fortunately, we have antioxidant defense systems that protect the body against free radical damage.

Antioxidants

Antioxidant Defense Systems

When oxygen appeared in the atmosphere of the earth, only those organisms that had developed antioxidant systems for protecting themselves against free radical damage survived and evolved. The antioxidant defense system in humans can be divided into three groups: (a) antioxidant enzymes made in the body, such as superoxide dismutase (SOD), catalase, and glutathione peroxidase; (b) antioxidants not made in the body and consumed principally through the diet (including vitamins A, C, and E; carotenoids; flavonoids; other polyphenols; and other antioxidants present in plants); and (c) antioxidants primarily made in the body but also consumed through the diet (primarily in meat and eggs) and in the form of supplements, including SH compounds (glutathione), coenzyme Q10, nicotinamide adenine dinucleotide (NADH), α-lipoic acid, and melatonin.

The antioxidant enzyme SOD requires manganese, copper, or zinc for its biological activity. Manganese-SOD is present in mitochondria, whereas copper-SOD and zinc-SOD are present in the cytoplasm and in the nucleus of the cell. They can destroy free radicals and hydrogen peroxide. Catalase needs iron for its biological activity, and it, too, destroys hydrogen peroxide in cells. Human tissue also contains glutathione peroxidase, which requires selenium for its biological activity and is responsible for removing hydrogen peroxide. Although iron, copper, and manganese are essential for the activities of antioxidant enzymes, a slight excess of free iron, copper, or manganese can amplify the production of free radicals and subsequently enhance the risk of various chronic diseases, including cancer.

Dietary Sources of Antioxidants

Carotenoids

There are more than six hundred carotenoids in plants, fruits, and vegetables, among them, xanthophyll, zeaxanthin, β-crytoxanthin, lutein, β-carotene, and lycopene. Beta-carotene has been studied extensively in laboratory experiments and in humans. At present, the roles of lutein, zeaxanthin, and lycopene in human health and cancer prevention also are being evaluated. Beta-carotene can be found in beets, broccoli, carrots, pumpkins, spinach, sweet potatoes, red cabbage, corn, cantaloupe, apricots, and mangoes. Tomatoes are the primary source of lycopene. Lutein predominates in spinach and marigold flowers. Paprika contains xanthophyll. All red and yellow fruits and vegetables have varying amounts of carotenoids.

Vitamin A

Liver, eggs, and milk are excellent sources of vitamin A.

Vitamin C

Many fruits contain vitamin C, among them, oranges, lemons, limes, pineapples, raspberries, strawberries, and grapefruit.

Vitamin E

Vegetable oils and nuts are a good source of vitamin E (predominantly, α-tocopherol); γ-, β-, and δ-tocopherols are also present in vegetable oils. Rice, oat bran, barley, and palm oil are rich in tocotrienols, another form of vitamin E.

Flavonoids, Polyphenols, and Other Plant-Derived Antioxidants

There are about five thousand flavonoids, which have been termed phytochemicals, in flowers, fruits, vegetables, and plants. Some of these substances under investigation include quercitin, geistein, and catechin. Commonly used herbs, such as ginkgo biloba and green tea, as well as green, leafy vegetables have flavonoids, polyphenols, and other antioxidants.

Commercially Available Antioxidants and Their Distribution in the Body

Carotenoids

Beta-carotene is one of more than six hundred carotenoids found in fruits, vegetables, and plants. It is commercially available in natural or synthetic forms. Preparations of natural β-carotene include more than one carotenoid. Synthetic preparations of β-carotene contain unknown impurities. A portion of ingested β-carotene becomes converted to vitamin A, and the remainder is distributed in the blood and tissues of the body. About twenty other carotenoids, including products of a variety of ingested carotenoids, also enter the blood and tissues. Beta-carotene is stored primarily in the eye and fatty tissue of the skin. In humans, the conversion of β-carotene to vitamin A does not occur if the body has sufficient stores of retinol (a form of vitamin A). Other carotenoids, such as lycopene and lutein, are sold commercially in natural but not synthetic forms. Some of these commercial preparations contain other components of carotenoids that are not usually mentioned on the label. A portion of ingested lycopene or lutein enters the blood and tissue. All carotenoids are considered fat-soluble antioxidants. Fat-soluble antioxidants should be taken with meals, so that they are more readily absorbed.

Vitamin A

Vitamin A is commercially available as retinyl acetate, retinol, retinyl palmitate, and retinoic acid and its analogues. Retinyl acetate (a stable form sold commercially) is converted to retinol (a form present in the body) in the intestine. Retinol then is converted to retinoic acid in cells. The latter form performs all the functions of vitamin A except in maintaining good vision. Retinoic acid and its analogues are used for experimental studies, because they are readily soluble in alcohol and thus enter cells easily. Vitamin A in blood takes the form of retinol and is stored in the liver as retinyl palmitate (a stable form sold commercially). The vitamin A product retinoic acid is stored in all body tissues. Vitamin A is a fat-soluble antioxidant.

Vitamin C

Vitamin C is sold commercially as ascorbic acid, sodium ascorbate (1 gram [g]of this type of vitamin C contains 124 mg of sodium), sodium ascorbate/minimum sodium (1 g of this type of vitamin C contains 62 mg of sodium), magnesium ascorbate, potassium ascorbate, calcium ascorbate, and time-release capsules containing ascorbic acid and vitamin C-ester. Vitamin C enters the blood as ascorbic acid and its product, dehydroascorbic acid.

Ascorbic acid supplements at high doses can cause upset stomach in some persons. Sodium ascorbate at high doses may increase the concentration of sodium in the urine, which can lead to chronic irritation of the bladder. Time-release capsules contain additional synthetic chemicals. Vitamin C-ester cannot function as vitamin C until the enzyme esterase removes the ester. For this reason, we recommend calcium ascorbate, which is buffered and is unlikely to produce adverse effects. All forms of vitamin C are water-soluble.

Vitamin E

Vitamin E is a term used for all tocopherols and tocotrienols possessing the biological activity of α-tocopherol. Both tocopherol and tocotrienol have α, β, γ, and δ forms. Alpha-tocopherol has the highest antioxidant activity, followed by β-, γ-, and δ-tocopherol. Synthetic vitamin E is referred to as the *dl* form; natural vitamin E is termed the *d* form. The common commercial variety of vitamin E is *d*- or *dl*-α-tocopherol. Other forms of vitamin E are *d*- or *dl*-α-tocopheryl acetate, -α-tocopheryl succinate, and -α-tocopheryl nicotinate. It has been assumed that these types of vitamin E are converted to α-tocopherol in the intestine and then are absorbed into the body. One study, however, reports that a portion of d-α-tocopheryl succinate can be absorbed as d-α-tocopheryl succinate and that it is not necessary that all vitamin E succinate be converted to α-tocopherol before absorption. Laboratory experiments have shown that the solvents of some vitamin E preparations are toxic (water-soluble forms) and should be avoided. Vitamin E should be taken both as d-α-tocopherol and d-α-tocopheryl succinate, since the latter has been found to be the most effective form of vitamin E in laboratory cell culture (in vitro) and in living beings (in vivo). Its effectiveness is based on the criteria of inhibition of tumor growth, induction of differentiation in some cancer cells, and gene regulation.

Flavonoids, Polyphenols, and Other Plant-Derived Antioxidants
Some flavonoids and other such antioxidants are sold commercially and are included in multiple vitamin preparations. They are fat-soluble.

Sulfhydryl Compounds
Sulfhydryl compounds are some of the most important antioxidants inside the cell and are commercially sold as N-acetylcysteine (NAC) and glutathione. In the body, N-acetyl is removed from NAC by the enzyme esterase, and then cysteine is used to make glutathione. When glutathione is taken orally, it is completely degraded in the intestinal tract; therefore, the consumption of glutathione will not increase glutathione levels in cells. NAC, an analogue of cysteine, is degraded only partially in the gut, and a portion of it will be available to cells to raise the intracellular level of glutathione. NAC is water-soluble.

Coenzyme Q10
Coenzyme Q10 is sold commercially as time-release or simple coenzyme Q10. It is absorbed in the body as coenzyme Q10.

Coenzyme Q10 is used by mitochondria to generate energy. It also acts as a weak antioxidant. A comparative study regarding the efficacy of time-release and regular forms has not been made. A portion of ingested coenzyme Q10 becomes available to cells to improve their functioning. This supplement is fat-soluble.

NADH

Only one form of NADH is sold commercially as a supplement. NADH is absorbed in the body as NADH. It is used by mitochondria to generate energy, and it acts as a weak antioxidant. NADH is water-soluble.

Alpha-Lipoic Acid and Melatonin

Both α-lipoic acid and melatonin are available commercially. Melatonin is sold in a time-release form. Both are soluble in alcohol. Alpha-lipoic acid raises the intracellular levels of glutathione and has strong cancer-fighting properties. Melatonin, a hormone produced by the pineal gland located in the brain, induces sleep, but it also acts as an antioxidant. It must be emphasized that melatonin should not be used as a routine supplement.

How to Store Antioxidants

Carotenoids

Most commercially sold carotenoids in solid form can be stored for a few years at room temperature, away from light. Beta-carotene in solution, however, degrades within a few days even in the cold and stored away from light.

Vitamin A

Crystal forms of retinol, retinoic acid, retinyl acetate, and retinyl palmitate can be stored at 4°C for several months. A solution of retinoic acid is stable at 4°C, stored away from the light, for several weeks.

Vitamin C

Vitamin C should not be stored in solution form, because it is easily destroyed within a few days. Crystal or tablet forms of vitamin C can be kept at room temperature, away from light, for a few years.

Vitamin E

Alpha-tocopherol, α-tocopheryl acetate, and α-tocopheryl succinate can be stored at room temperature, away from light, for a few years. A solution of α-tocopheryl succinate is stable for several months at 4°C if kept away from the light.

Flavonoids, Polyphenols, and Other Plant-Derived Antioxidants

These supplements are stable in solid form at room temperature, away from the light, for a few years.

Sulfhydryl Compounds, Coenzyme Q10, and NADH

These antioxidants in solid form are stable at room temperature, away from the light, for a few years. The solutions of these compounds are stable at 4°C away from the light for several months.

Alpha-Lipoic Acid and Melatonin

Alpha-lipoic acid can be stored at room temperature away from the light for a few years. Melatonin can be stored in the refrigerator for a year or more.

Can Antioxidants Be Destroyed During Cooking?

Carotenoids

At least a portion of β-carotene is destroyed during cooking. Some carotenoids, especially lutein and lycopene, are not harmed significantly by cooking. In fact, their bioavailability improves when they are derived from a cooked or extracted preparation, for example, from tomato sauce in the case of lycopene.

Vitamin A
Routine cooking does not destroy vitamin A, but slow heating over a long period of time may reduce its potency. Canning and prolonged cold storage also may diminish vitamin A's activity. The vitamin A content of fortified milk powder substantially declines after two years.

Vitamin C
Freezing, thawing, and cold storage of solutions of vitamin C lessen its potency. Vitamin C is destroyed during cooking, through oxidation.

Vitamin E
Food processing, frying, and freezing destroy vitamin E. The vitamin E content of fortified milk powder is unaffected over a two-year period.

Sulfhydryl Compounds, Coenzyme Q10, and NADH
Some SH compounds, NADH, and coenzyme Q10 can be partially degraded during cooking.

Alpha-Lipoic Acid and Melatonin
Alpha lipoic acid and melatonin can be partially destroyed during cooking.

Why We Need Micronutrient Supplements
Adequate amounts of micronutrients (such as vitamins A, C, and E; carotenoids; flavonoids and other poylphenols; SH compounds; coenzyme Q10; and NADH) are essential for growth and development of the human body. A deficiency in one of these antioxidants can have serious effects on health. The constant use of oxygen in the body generates large amounts of free radicals, which are harmful chemicals. Free radicals also are produced during infection and during the normal metabolism of certain substances. Specific metal ions, such as iron, copper, and manganese, in combination with molecules like vitamin C and

uric acid can generate large amounts of free radicals. Antioxidants can destroy such excessive quantities of free radicals in the body and also can stimulate the immune system, prevent the formation of harmful chemicals during digestion of food, reduce the frequency of mutations (changes in genes) caused by environmental and dietary toxins, and enhance the repair of damage brought about by radiation and chemicals. They also regulate gene activity in cancer cells in a way that helps curtail the growth of tumor cells. It must be emphasized, however, that many of the actions of antioxidants on cancer cells are not due to their antioxidative properties but rather to their role in regulating gene activity. Thus, maintaining adequate amounts of antioxidants in the body is vital to optimal health and disease prevention.

The RDA (recommended dietary allowance) value for each micronutrient has been established (see chapter 7), and these values are considered sufficient for preventing deficiencies and for allowing normal growth and development. These values may not be enough for optimal health and for disease prevention and treatment, however. In addition, vitamin E, vitamin A (for some vegetarians), SH compounds, coenzyme Q10, NADH, and vitamin C may not be obtainable in adequate amounts from one's diet alone though flavonoids and other polyphenols are adequately represented in the diet. We believe that moderate supplementation of certain micronutrients, including antioxidants, is essential. The dosage, type, and number of micronutrients needed for optimal health and disease prevention or treatment depend on a person's age, sex, type of disease, disease risk levels (low risk or high risk), and disease stage (early or advanced stage). These topics are addressed in chapters 5 and 6.

How Much of Each Antioxidant Do We Absorb and Retain?

Beta-carotene

Only about 10 percent of ingested β-carotene is absorbed from the small intestine. Among vegetarians who do not eat eggs or dairy products, most β-carotene is converted to retinol, whereas among non-vegetarians (who have sufficient stores of vitamin A) such conversion does not take place. The turnover of β-carotene in the blood is slow; therefore, it can be taken as a supplement once or twice per day to maintain a relatively constant level of this nutrient.

Vitamin A

Only about 10 to 20 percent of ingested vitamin A is absorbed from the small intestine. Normal cells characteristically do not take up more than they need to function. Liver cells are an exception. Retinyl acetate is converted to retinol in the intestine. Retinol is converted further to retinoic acid in cells; however, most of the body's vitamin A is stored in the liver as retinyl palmitate. Since retinol reaches its maximum level in the blood 3 to 6 hours after ingestion of vitamin A and drops to a basal level in about 12 hours, vitamin A should be taken twice a day (once in the morning and once in the evening) to maintain constant levels.

Vitamin C

Absorption of ingested vitamin C varies from 20 to 80 percent, depending upon the dose. If one consumes 200 to 500 mg, only 50 percent (100 to 250 mg) will be absorbed from the intestine. To reduce the formation of cancer-causing substances in the stomach and intestine, a certain amount of unabsorbed vitamin C may be useful. Once absorbed, vitamin C is rapidly distributed throughout the body. As with vitamin A, normal cells do not take up more vitamin C than they need to function. Since vitamin C is degraded rapidly in the body, the maintenance of constant blood levels may require taking vitamin C at least two times per day.

Vitamin E

Vitamin E can be taken as both α-tocopherol and α-tocopheryl succinate. A portion of α-tocopheryl succinate is converted to α-tocopherol in the intestine before absorption, but a portion also is absorbed without degradation. About 20 percent of ingested α-tocopherol is absorbed from the small intestine and is distributed quickly throughout the body. As with vitamins A and C, normal cells do not take up greater amounts of α-tocopherol or α-tocopheryl succinate than they need. Since the maximum levels of α-tocopherol in the blood appear 4 to 6 hours after it is ingested and drop to a basal level in about 12 hours, the maintenance of constant blood levels of vitamin E requires taking it twice per day (morning and evening).

Flavonoids, Polyphenols, and Other Plant-Derived Antioxidants

These antioxidants are consumed in large quantities (grams) through the diet; for this reason, supplementation of a few milligrams in pills is not recommended.

Sulfhydryl Compounds

Sulfhydryl compounds are fairly stable in cells. One of the most common of these compounds is glutathione. Increased oxidative stress can diminish SH levels inside the cells. Glutathione cannot be taken orally, however, because it is completely degraded in the human intestine. Therefore, NAC, which is degraded only partially in the gut and which raises the intracellular levels of glutathione following oral administration, is recommended. Taking a supplement once a day may be sufficient to maintain a constant cellular level of glutathione. It should be emphasized that this antioxidant is not recommended for all persons. (See chapters 5 and 6 for details.)

Coenzyme Q10 and NADH

Coenzyme Q10 and NADH are made in the human body. Their cellular levels are relatively constant unless cells are damaged. Various preparations of coenzyme Q10 and only one preparation of NADH are available commercially. The absorption of coenzyme Q10 from the intestinal tract varies, depending upon the preparation. The absorption of NADH has not been studied in humans, but the oral intake of NADH has been shown to have beneficial effects in such neurodegenerative conditions as Alzheimer's disease and Parkinson's disease. This suggests that orally administered NADH can enter the brain. Taking coenzyme Q10 and NADH once a day may maintain constant cellular levels of these antioxidants, but they are not recommended for everyone. (See chapters 5 and 6 for details.)

Alpha-Lipoic Acid and Melatonin

Alpha-lipoic acid is made in the body and is absorbed from the intestinal tract and rapidly distributed into various tissues. Its product, dihydrolipoic acid, also acts as an antioxidant. Both substances remove metals from the body. Lipoic acid is not recommended for everyone. (See chapters 5 and 6 for detailed recommendations.) Melatonin also is absorbed from the intestinal tract, but it is degraded rapidly in the body. This hormone is not recommended as a supplement except for people who have occasional sleeping problems.

Which Antioxidant Supplements Should We Take? How Much and How Often?

At this time, the doses of antioxidants imparting the greatest benefit to human health and maximum reduction of cancer risk are unknown. Nevertheless, some studies have estimated that about 40 percent of all Americans take micronutrients on a regular basis. Many people with cancer or other illnesses take these supplements in some form, without their doctors' approval.

When one talks with people who are taking micronutrients on the advice of a salesperson at a vitamin store, health-related magazines, and books or television reporting, it becomes evident that they are doing so without reference to any scientific rationale. Furthermore, the makers of most preparations of multiple vitamins with minerals have not given adequate attention to the doses, type, and chemical form of antioxidants or the appropriate minerals. For example, most of the commercially sold multiple antioxidant formulas with minerals include iron, copper, or manganese—or all three. It is known that iron, copper, or manganese, when combined with vitamin C, generate free radicals. In addition, in the presence of antioxidants these minerals are absorbed better from the intestinal tract and thus increase the body's stores of these minerals. Enhanced iron stores in the body have been associated with many human chronic diseases, including cancer, heart disease, and neurological diseases. Therefore, the addition of iron, copper, or manganese to any multiple antioxidant preparation has no scientific merit in terms of ensuring optimal health or preventing disease. In cases where a person has iron-deficiency anemia, a short-term iron supplement is essential, until the anemia is cured.

Many commercially sold multiple antioxidant preparations contain heavy metals, such as boron, vanadium, and molybdenum. Sufficient amounts of these metals are obtained from the diet. The daily consumption of excess amounts of these metals over a long period of time can be neurotoxic. Many commercial preparations of antioxidants also include inositol, methionine, and choline in varying doses (30 to 60 mg). Such doses of these nutrients serve no useful purpose, because 400 to 1,000 mg are obtained daily from the diet. Paraaminobenzoic acid (PABA) is present in some multiple vitamin preparations. PABA has no biologic function in mammalian cells. In addition, it blocks the antibacterial effects of sulfonamides. Therefore, patients taking sulfonamides and a multiple antioxidant containing PABA may experience diminished effectiveness of the drug.

Commercially sold multiple antioxidant preparations often contain NAC or α-lipoic acid. These nutrients increase glutathione levels in the cells. Glutathione is a powerful antioxidant that protects both normal and cancer cells against radiation damage. The consumption of antioxidant preparations containing NAC or α-lipoic acid by cancer patients undergoing radiation therapy could be harmful, since glutathione will obviate the desired effects of radiation on cancer cells.

The addition of both β-carotene and vitamin A to any multiple vitamin preparation is essential, because β-carotene not only acts as a parent of vitamin A but also has important biological functions that vitamin A does not. For example, β-carotene increases the activity of the connexin gene, which produces a gap junction protein that is necessary for maintaining the normal shape of cells. Other carotenoids, such as lycopene and lutein, are also important for health, but they can be obtained from a diet rich in tomato (lycopene), spinach (lutein), and paprika (xanthophylls, including lutein) in amounts that are much higher than those that can be found in supplements. Therefore, the addition of a few milligrams of lycopene and lutein and other xanthophylls to any multiple vitamin preparation serves no useful purpose for maintenance of health or disease prevention.

Two forms of vitamin E, *d*-α-tocopherol (present in the body) and *d*-α-tocopheryl succinate, should be present in a multiple antioxidant preparation, because α-tocopheryl succinate is the most effective form of vitamin E inside the cells, while α-tocopherol can readily act as an antioxidant in the intestinal tract and in the extracellular environment of the body. Alpha-tocopherol (at doses of 20 to 60 mcg per milliliter) can stimulate the immune system, but β-, γ-, and δ forms at similar doses can inhibit the immune system. This effect may not be related to their antioxidant action, because they are less effective than α-tocopherol. For this reason, supplementation with β-, γ-, and δ-tocopherol is not recommended. Similarly, tocotrienols inhibit cholesterol synthesis; therefore they cannot be used as supplements for optimal health. Prolonged inhibition of cholesterol synthesis in healthy persons with normal cholesterol levels may cause illness. Cholesterol is necessary to maintain normal functioning of all cells, particularly brain cells.

Vitamin C is most suitable taken in the form of calcium ascorbate, because it is not acidic and doesn't cause upset stomach (as ascorbic acid can). The addition of potassium ascorbate and magnesium ascorbate to any multiple vitamin preparation is unnecessary. Adequate of amounts of B vitamins (two to three times the RDA) and appropriate minerals, such as selenium, zinc, and chromium, should be included in any multiple antioxidant preparation. (B vitamins have no relevance to cancer prevention. For this reason, we do not discuss them at length here.)

It is impossible to recommend an appropriate multiple antioxidant supplement that can be useful to everyone, irrespective of age, sex, general health, and disease status. It appears to be more rational to take one basic multiple antioxidant product that contains all the nutrients necessary for optimal health and then supplement it with additional antioxidants and other nutrients based on individual factors. This issue is discussed in chapter 5.

Do We Need Supplementary Antioxidants for Optimal Health or Disease Prevention and Treatment?

A balanced diet may be sufficient for normal growth, but supplemental micronutrients, including antioxidants, are important for maintaining optimal health and for disease prevention and treatment. One would have difficulty eating fresh fruits and vegetables daily in the amounts and at the rates that maintain ideal levels of β-carotene and vitamins A, C, and E in the blood. It is necessary to take supplemental antioxidants in addition to eating a balanced diet. An advantage of taking supplemental antioxidants is that one can do so at the most appropriate time to prevent the formation of cancer-causing agents and limit their carcinogenic effects, such as just before eating food containing nitrites or other cancer-causing substances.

Even some scientists believe that it is enough to eat a balanced diet to maintain health and prevent disease, but many studies suggest that most foods have naturally occurring toxic as well as protective substances. A balanced diet alone may not prevent disease. While a balanced diet is better than junk food and will protect against vitamin deficiency, the main problems with the concept of such a diet are that it is too general and that interpretation can vary markedly from one person to another. Some people believe that a daily intake of one apple, one carrot, one orange, a few other fresh vegetables, a little meat, and some carbohydrates constitutes a balanced diet; other people define a balanced diet completely differently, with more or less of these individual foods. Even if a balanced diet is defined more precisely, the same balanced diet cannot be applied to all regions of the world, because dietary and environmental levels of cancer-causing substances vary markedly from one region to another.

Thus, supplemental antioxidants may be necessary to lower the risk of cancer.

With respect to cancer prevention, it is vital to ingest certain antioxidants at the right time; otherwise, their possible effectiveness against cancer is minimized. For example, if taken immediately before eating nitrite-rich food, vitamins C and E can moderate the formation of nitrosamines in the stomach. Taking these vitamins a few hours after such a meal may not be as effective. Furthermore, studies have shown that levels of fecal mutagens (a possible source of cancer) in people who regularly eat meat are much higher than in vegetarians. Vitamins C and E have been found to reduce the levels of mutagens in the feces. For this reason, these vitamins should be taken just before or immediately after eating meat. (Consult chapters 5 and 6 for specifics.)

The intake of absolute amounts of antioxidants may not be an important issue in cancer prevention. Instead, the relative levels of cancer-causing substances present in the diet and the environment and the relative levels of anticancer micronutrients, such as antioxidants and selenium, present in the body are crucial in determining the potential risk for cancer. Consequently, increased consumption of cancer-causing substances and a high level of exposure to such agents in the environment would require a proportional increase in available anticancer micronutrients, which can be supplied by supplemental micronutrients.

As we pointed out earlier, all types of diets, including those that are defined as balanced diets, contain both toxic and protective substances. Some toxic agents, such as pesticides, are synthetic, whereas others are found in nature. The risk of chronic illness, including cancer, may depend upon the relative consumption of protective versus toxic substances. If the daily intake of protective substances is higher than that of toxic agents, the risk of chronic illness would be lower. Since we know very little about the relative levels of toxic and protective substances in any diet, we cannot know whether we are consuming higher levels of protective substances compared with toxic ones. To ensure a higher intake of protective agents, it is necessary to take a daily supplement of micronutrients, including antioxidants.

Risks of Taking Micronutrients

The risk of taking micronutrients depends upon doses, forms, frequency of ingestion and duration of consumption as well as whether they are taken as a single agent or as part of a multiple micronutrient preparation. It is well established that when an individual antioxidant is oxidized, it can act as a free radical. For example, when vitamin C is consumed alone at high doses, it can act as both an antioxidant and pro-oxidant. This was clearly established in a recent study in which vitamin C was found to lower levels of the oxidized DNA base guanosine (a form of DNA damage) in human lymphocytes (a type of blood cell), suggesting that vitamin C protects DNA from oxidative injury. In the same publication, it was reported that vitamin C enhances levels of the oxidized DNA base adenine (another form of DNA damage), indicating that the same dose of vitamin C intensifies oxidative injury of DNA. Vitamin C in combination with other antioxidants is unlikely to produce such a dual effect. One study has suggested that taking synthetic β-carotene alone, at a daily dose of 25 mg, can increase the risk of lung cancer among groups of people who are at higher-than-average risk of lung cancer, such as men who are heavy smokers.

Beta-carotene

There is no known toxic effect of β-carotene in doses up to 50 mg per day in normal human subjects. Bronzing of the skin may appear after oral ingestion of β-carotene at 100 mg per day or more over a few months. Deposits of β-carotene pigment are found in the eye after long-term consumption of high doses of β-carotene. Excessive pigment deposit can harm the eye. These changes are reversible upon discontinuation of the supplement. The other carotenoids, such as lutein and lycopene, are relatively nontoxic at oral doses up to 50 mg per day.

Vitamin A

Liver toxicity and skin reactions have been noted after oral ingestion of 50,000 IU per day of vitamin A over a year or more. Some of these changes are reversible when the vitamin is discontinued. Liver toxicity can be irreversible. Up to 10,000 IU of vitamin A, taken orally and divided into two doses per day, is unlikely to produce major toxic effects in a normal adult. Pregnant women should avoid taking more than 5,000 IU of vitamin A, because higher doses may have adverse effects on the fetus. Retinoic acid and other derivatives of vitamin A should not be consumed orally for general health maintenance, because of the toxic effects of these compounds at relatively low doses.

Vitamin C

In most healthy people, doses of vitamin C up to 10 g per day taken orally will not produce any detectable toxic effects. In certain diseases involving iron metabolism (hemochromatosis) or copper metabolism (Wilson disease) or resulting from excessive exposure to manganese (Parkinsonian syndrome), excessive consumption of vitamin C may be harmful, because vitamin C in combination with iron, copper, or manganese, in the presence of oxygen, generates free radicals. According to many studies, up to 2 g of vitamin C, taken orally and divided into at least two doses per day, is unlikely to cause any serious side effects in a normal adult. There is no scientific evidence that vitamin C supplementation at high doses raises the risk of kidney stones or gout in most normal people. As mentioned previously, increased urinary excretion of oxalic acid in people taking high doses of vitamin C has been interpreted to mean that this vitamin may increase the risk of kidney stones, since enhanced excretion of oxalic acid also is found in most patients with kidney stones. These could be the result of independent biochemical reactions, however, and the two events may not necessarily be linked. There were no documented cases of an elevated incidence of kidney stones among any study group taking high doses of vitamin C.

Vitamin E
In a large human trial that enrolled nine thousand adults, a daily oral intake of 3,000 IU per day of α-tocopherol acetate for eleven years did not produce any detectable major side effects, though isolated cases of fatigue, skin reactions, and upset stomach have been reported after ingestion of high doses (more than 1,000 IU daily) of vitamin E for a prolonged period of time. High doses of vitamin E (2,000 IU daily) can cause a blood-clotting defect, which is reversible after administration of vitamin K. According to many studies, up to 400 IU of vitamin E taken orally, divided into two doses per day, is not likely to have any significant toxic effects in a normal adult.

Flavonoids, Polyphenols, and Other Plant-Derived Antioxidants
Although these antioxidants have no known toxicity, the adverse consequences of high doses of these compounds have not been evaluated in humans.

Sulfhydryl Compounds
N-acetylcysteine is commonly used to increase intracellular levels of glutathione. An oral dose of 800 mg or more over a period 6 months or more can amplify the urinary excretion of zinc, which can induce zinc deficiency unless a zinc supplement is taken. A dose of up to 500 mg, with zinc supplementation, is considered safe.

Coenzyme Q10 and NADH

Oral doses up to 300 mg of coenzyme Q10 have been given to patients with breast cancer without significant apparent toxicity. Similar high doses of coenzyme Q10 have been used in the treatment of advanced cardiac disease without adverse effects. NADH has been administered at an oral dose of 10 mg per day or more for the treatment of neurodegenerative diseases, without any deleterious effects.

Alpha-Lipoic Acid and Melatonin

Alpha-lipoic acid acts as a metal chelator; for this reason, long-term consumption at high doses may induce metal deficiency. Some people can suffer allergic reactions, and diabetic patients might experience hypoglycemia. Melatonin is thought to be fairly benign, but the long-term effects of supplemental melatonin at low doses (1 to 10 mg/day and typically 3 mg/day) are not known.

Protease Inhibitors

Protease inhibitors are found in large amounts in soybeans. They inhibit the activities of cellular enzymes called proteases, which destroy proteins in the cells. A precise balance between the rate of formation and destruction of protein must be maintained in the cells for their optimal function. Even in moderate amounts, protease inhibitors (taken as a supplement) can disturb this balance and produce all sorts of toxic effects. Some laboratory experiments suggest that protease inhibitors, such as antipain, block cancer formation by radiation and also the action of tumor promoters. The significance of protease inhibitors in reducing the risk of cancer in human beings is being evaluated. Meanwhile, the value of consuming large amounts of soybeans and products derived from soybeans (e.g., tofu) is in doubt. Protease inhibitors are not recommended for consumption as a supplement, and soybeans should be eaten only in moderation.

Selenium

Among minerals, the results of animal studies seem to indicate that selenium is a potent anticancer agent. An antioxidant enzyme, glutathione peroxidase, requires selenium in order to exert its antioxidant action. Selenium in combination with vitamin E is more effective than either nutrient taken alone. Analyses of dietary intake of selenium and cancer incidence have shown that the mineral also may lower the risk of cancer, particularly prostate cancer, in human beings. Certain metals, such as lead, cadmium, arsenic, mercury, and silver, block the action of selenium.

It is a common belief that high doses of zinc are important for maintaining health, but this may not be true with respect to cancer prevention. Recent laboratory experiments have shown that high doses of zinc block the action of selenium. One has to be careful about taking excessive amounts of zinc (more than 20 mg per day from diet and supplements combined) while taking selenium. Diets rich in protein and unsaturated fats have been shown to increase the selenium requirements of the body. These studies suggest that in terms of gaining the greatest cancer-preventing benefits of selenium, a person should eat a diet low in those metals that block the action of selenium and one that provides adequate but not immoderate amounts of zinc, protein, and unsaturated fats.

Commercial preparations of selenium include inorganic selenium (sodium selenite) and various organic compounds of selenium. Some studies have reported that sodium selenite is not absorbed adequately, whereas organic selenium, including yeast-selenium and seleno-L-methionine, is absorbed very well. For this reason, organic selenium is considered best for human consumption. The optimal doses of selenium in terms of its health benefits are unknown. In the United States, the average dietary intake of selenium is 125 to 150 mcg per day. The RDA of selenium for adults is 55 to 70 mcg per day. About 250 to 300 mcg of selenium a day (through diet and supplements) has been reported to be helpful in preventing cancer. If an average person consumes 125 to 150 mcg of selenium each day, a supplement of 100 mcg each day is unlikely to give rise to any major side effects. Animal studies suggest that 2 to 3 mcg per g of diet (twenty to thirty times the human RDA) every day may produce adverse effects. The window of safety for selenium intake is very narrow. A total daily intake (diet and supplement) of 500 mcg or more of selenium may be toxic to humans. Toxic effects include dry skin and cataract formation.

Concluding Remarks

Free radicals are highly damaging chemicals that are produced constantly in the human body. They are generated during the use of oxygen, in the course of bacterial infection, and in the context of the normal metabolism of various compounds in the body. There are several types of free radicals, the levels of which can vary from one organ to another. We have developed antioxidant systems to protect against the damaging effects of free radicals. Some antioxidants are made in the body, whereas others are consumed through a diet containing fruits and vegetables. The biological half-life (time needed to remove a substance from the body by half) of most antioxidants is 6 to 12 hours; therefore, they should be taken twice a day to maintain a constant level of these nutrients in the body. Most antioxidants are sensitive to light and should be stored in the dark. They are stable at room temperature.

Certain antioxidants can be toxic at high doses. A general preparation of multiple micronutrients should not contain all antioxidants, because some are harmful under certain conditions. For example, NAC and α-lipoic acid protect cancer cells against radiation damage; for this reason, cancer patients undergoing chemotherapy or radiation therapy should not take these antioxidants. Consumption of a high-fiber diet is very important for cancer prevention, because such a diet eliminates potential mutagens and carcinogens from the gut and generates high levels of butyric acid, a powerful anticancer agent. A low-fat diet is equally important for optimal health.

3 The Facts about Cancer

The human genome (genetic material of the human body) contains about fifty thousand genes, but only about five thousand to ten thousand genes are active. This genome sustains about ten thousand mutations (changes in gene activity) per day. It is exposed constantly to mutagens (agents altering gene activity) and carcinogens (agents causing cancer by altering specific gene activity) from environmental, dietary, and lifestyle-related factors. One of the consequences of such exposure is the development of cancer. Most cancers occur spontaneously; however, a few are hereditary. Familial tumors often arise at an early age, but spontaneously occurring tumors can develop at any age. Only some cancers are related to gender, such as prostate cancer in men and ovarian and cervical cancer in women. Some cancers develop more commonly at certain ages, such as colon cancer in older people and neuroblastoma (a childhood cancer of embryonic nerve cells) and Wilms tumor (a tumor of the kidney) in younger people. Most cancers, however, can appear at any age.

There is also regional variation in the type and incidence of cancer. In the industrialized nations of the West, such as the United States and Europe, the predominant types include breast, colon, and prostate cancer. In the industrialized nations of the East, such as Japan, the incidence of breast cancer is low, but the incidence of gastric and liver cancer is high. In developing countries, such as India, the Middle East, and China, the incidence of gastric cancer, liver cancer, and cervical cancer is high. The incidence of lung cancer is high in many areas of the world, because of similar smoking habits. In the U.S. population of about 300 million, about 1.2 million new cases of cancer are detected every year, and about six hundred thousand people die each year of cancer. This would indicate that some form of cancer will develop in one of every four people during his or her lifetime.

What Are Cancer Cells?

Cancer cells divide like normal cells but, unlike normal cells, which undergo differentiation and death, they continue to divide without restriction and invade distant organs in the body. The process of invading distant organs is called metastasis. When normal cells are grown outside the body in laboratory petri dishes, a procedure known as tissue culture or cell culture, they have a limited life span, and all eventually die even when they have nutrients and space to grow. In this sense, normal cells can be considered mortal, whereas cancer cells are immortal. Cancer cells will continue to grow in tissue culture dishes indefinitely, provided sufficient nutrients and space are available. Cancer can arise in any organ that contains dividing cells (e.g., bone marrow, skin, intestine, breast, lung, prostate) or that has cells that normally do not divide but that will divide if properly stimulated (e.g., liver cells and glial cells in the brain).

Cancer is the common term used for all malignant tumors. The term *tumor* originally referred to swelling due to inflammation, but it now refers to both malignant and benign growths. The growth of all cancer cells depends upon the host for nutrition and vascular supply. Some endocrine tumors, such as certain ovarian, breast, and prostate cancers, also use sex hormones for their growth.

Classification of Tumors

Tumors can be classified into two major categories: benign tumors and malignant tumors. Benign tumor cells divide abnormally and form a mass but do not metastasize. Examples of benign tumors are polyps in the colon, adenomas of the thyroid, leiomyomas (fibroid tumors of the uterus), and fibroadenomas of the breast. Most benign tumors do not become cancerous. Rarely, however, cancer can arise in a benign tumor. For example, leiomyosarcoma can develop in a leiomyoma. Malignant tumors are those that can metastasize (spread) to distant organs. If they arise from mesenchymal tissue (such as connective tissue, blood, bone, and cartilage), they are called sarcomas. A few examples of sarcoma are fibrosarcoma and liposarcoma. If malignant tumors arise from epithelial cells (that is, cells that form a membranous tissue that covers surfaces or lines cavities of the body), they are called carcinomas. Adenocarcinoma of the lung and squamous cell carcinoma of the skin fall into this category. Other types of malignancies include melanoma (cancer of pigment-producing cells called melanocytes) and lymphoma (cancer of white blood cells). Most human tumors are of epithelial origin. Most malignant tumors have the capacity to metastasize, except for glioblastoma (a brain tumor) and basal cell carcinoma (a skin tumor). Different tumors spread through distinct pathways. Some tumors migrate to various organs through the lymphatic system and others through the blood vessels. The liver and lungs are common sites for metastases.

Major Warning Signs and Symptoms of Cancer

General: Weakness, fatigue, and significant weight loss

Breast cancer: Persistent lump, bloody discharge from the nipple, ulcer that does not heal, retraction of the nipple, dimpling of the skin

Lung cancer: Persistent cough, coughing up blood, chest pain

Cervical cancer: Spotting of blood after intercourse, painful intercourse, foul discharge from the vagina

Skin cancer: Increase in size, ulceration, or change in color of mole; non-healing and persistent ulcer

Rectal and colon cancer: Alternating diarrhea and constipation, bloody discharge in the stool associated with weight loss

Bone cancer: Prolonged pain in bones without any injury, with or without swelling

Testicular cancer: Persistent, firm swelling in the testis, usually without pain

Hodgkin disease: Firm and painless enlargement of the lymph nodes, fever, excess sweating, fatigue

Leukemia: Weakness, loss of appetite, bone and joint pain, fever, lymph node swelling

How Do Normal Cells Become Cancerous?

In a general sense, it is believed that when normal dividing cells accumulate several genetic defects (mutations or altered gene expression), they become cancer cells. Specific genes responsible for the change of normal cells to cancer cells have not been identified. The process of cancer can be divided into two phases: the tumor-initiating phase and the tumor-promoting phase. During the initiating phase, cells divide abnormally, forming a mass. When normal cells suffer damage in a specific gene, they divide abnormally but do not spread to distant organs. An example of such abnormally growing masses are polyps in the colon. Agents that can initiate this process of carcinogenesis are called *tumor initiators*. These abnormal cells continue to grow without becoming cancerous for several years. During the promoting phase, when specific gene mutations occur in abnormally dividing cells, they become cancerous. Agents that cause tumor promotion are called *tumor promoters*. High doses of tumor initiators are sufficient to produce cancer; low doses of tumor initiators cannot cause cancer unless they are helped by tumor promoters. Even high doses of tumor promoters alone generally do not give rise to cancer. Normal cells also contain sets of genes that are called *anti-oncogenes,* or tumor-suppressor genes. The products (proteins) of anti-oncogenes prevent normal cells from becoming cancer cells. Several tumor-suppressor genes have been identified, among them p53, Rb, and p21.

Human beings seldom are exposed to high doses of tumor initiators or promoters, but they are exposed frequently to low doses of these cancer-causing substances. Cancer-initiated events may remain dormant for ten to thirty years or more; when further specific genetic changes occur during the promotion phase, they cause cancer. Laboratory experiments have shown that the combined influence of two initiators is more effective in producing cancer than the influence of individual agents acting alone. Some commonly known tumor initiators and tumor promoters are listed below. Most of them are found in the environment and diet. The percentage of cancer deaths among men and women differ, depending upon the form of cancer (Table 1).

Commonly Known Tumor Initiators

Nitrosamine

7,12-Dimethylbenz(a)anthracene

Benzo(a)pyrene

Asbestos

Ultraviolet radiation

Tobacco smoke

Polychlorinated biphenyl

Diethylstilbestrol

Aflatoxin

Polyvinyl chloride

Pesticides (malathion, parathion, kepone, DDT)

Ionizing radiation (X rays and gamma rays)

Some chemotherapeutic agents

Tar

Dioxin

Commonly Known Tumor Promoters

Saccharine

Excess fat, proteins, or carbohydrates

12-*O*-tetradecanoylphorbol-13-acetate (found in coal tar)

High temperatures (43–45°C, or 109.4–111°F)

Certain hormones, such as estrogen

Extract of unburned tobacco

Tobacco smoke condensate

Surface-active agents (sodium lauryl sulfate), found in
toothpaste and chewing gum, for example

Iodoacetic acid

Phenobarbital

**Table 1 — Percentages of Deaths from Cancer of Different
Parts of the Body in Men and Women**

Cancer Site	Men	Women
Lung	34	16
Colon and rectum	12	15
Prostate	10	—
Breast	—	19
Female reproductive organs (ovary, uterus, and cervix)	—	11

About three hundred thousand Americans have prostate cancer, and in 1997 forty thousand deaths were attributed to this disease. Approximately five hundred thousand new cases of skin cancer are detected every year. Colorectal cancer is second only to lung cancer as the most common cause of death from cancer. About 130,000 cases of colon and rectal cancer were diagnosed in 1999, and fifty-six thousand people died of these diseases. Breast cancer is the most common cancer in women and the third most common cancer in the world. The annual incidence of breast cancer is about 182,000 cases.

Interpretation of Laboratory Data for Human Carcinogenesis

In laboratory experiments involving cells growing in dishes or using animals, a single tumor initiator, alone or in combination with a tumor promoter, is commonly used for the study of carcinogenesis. Therefore, the dose of these agents needed to cause cancer is high. The relevance of these observations to humans is often ignored on the ground that humans are never exposed to such high levels of tumor initiators or tumor promoters. This attitude is without scientific merit, because humans are exposed to many tumor initiators and tumor promoters at very low doses. Laboratory experiments have shown that these potential carcinogens interact with each other synergistically to produce tumors; for this reason, the significance of laboratory data on high doses of chemical carcinogens should not be ignored, and every effort must be made to reduce exposure to all carcinogens identified by laboratory experiments.

Interpretation of Human Carcinogenesis Studies

Epidemiologic experiments are the only tool available to study the association of potential carcinogens on human cancer. These experiments represent a powerful and useful method for establishing an association between potential carcinogens and the risk of cancer. It is misleading and incorrect, however, to interpret epidemiological studies to mean that a potential carcinogen identified by these experiments actually causes cancer in humans. The epidemiological findings must be confirmed by laboratory experiments on human cells before such potential carcinogens are designated as human carcinogens.

Concluding Remarks

Cancer remains one of the major health concerns of the U.S. population. One of every four people will develop some form of cancer during his or her lifetime. Although many gene defects play a part in human carcinogenesis, the genes that initiate cancer formation have not been identified. Studies are in progress to single out such genes in human cells. Nevertheless, many tumor initiators and tumor promoters have been detected, and thus we can work to limit our exposure to these carcinogens. If they are not properly performed and interpreted, epidemiological studies can cause confusion among the public concerning which factors play significant roles in causing cancer or increasing the risk of cancer.

4 Mutagens and Carcinogens in the Environment, Lifestyle, and Diet

In order to develop a rational strategy for cancer prevention in humans, it is essential to identify sources of carcinogens and mutagens in the environment, lifestyle, and diet. More than 95 percent of all human cancers have some components of risk associated with these factors. Exposure to carcinogens also occurs in the workplace and during the diagnosis and treatment of cancer.

Environmental Factors in Carcinogenesis

Ionizing Radiation (X Rays and Gamma Rays)

One environmental source of ionizing radiation is cosmic radiation(gamma rays), the levels of which increase at higher altitudes. For example, the background level of cosmic radiation in Denver, a city located at an elevation of 5,500 feet (one mile) is two times higher than that found in New York City, which is at sea level. The environment near uranium mines contains radon gas, a by-product of radioactive uranium. Nuclear testing in the past also has contributed to elevated levels of ionizing radiation in the atmosphere, but this level of exposure is minimal compared with that from cosmic radiation. Flying in planes at high altitudes has been cited as posing a risk, but it represents an insignificant increase in radiation exposure.

Ionizing radiation (X rays) is commonly used to diagnose human diseases, and radiation therapy is often given to treat cancer. Such radiation, however, also can cause cancer. The minimum radiation dose (one exposure and whole body) needed to induce leukemia in adults is about 0.2 gray (Gy, unit of absorbed dose of radiation). Just 0.01 Gy is equal to the radiation exposure of approximately thirty-three chest X-ray films.) In human fetuses, any amount of radiation can induce leukemia. Repeated exposure to small doses of radiation is more likely to cause leukemia than a large single dose. Most forms of leukemia appear within ten years from the time of radiation exposure.

The minimum dose of radiation needed to give rise to breast cancer is about 0.01 Gy. Breast tissue is more sensitive to irradiation during pregnancy. The minimum dose of radiation needed to produce thyroid cancer is about 0.07 Gy. Women are approximately two times more sensitive than men; Jewish women seem to be about seventeen times more sensitive than non-Jewish women. The reasons for these differences are unknown at this time. The time period between exposure to radiation and cancer development can vary from five years to more than thirty-five years. Doses typically used in radiation therapy (a total of 30 to 40 Gy, given at 2 Gy per treatment and 10 Gy per week) can induce cancer in most organs five to thirty years after the completion of radiation therapy.

Some laboratory studies suggest that the combination of ionizing radiation and chemical carcinogens is nine times more likely to cause cancer than are the individual agents alone. Ionizing radiation also promotes virus-induced cancer formation in laboratory experiments. Since there is no radiation dose known to be "safe," continuous efforts must be made to minimize exposure. No one should be exposed to extra radiation, unless it is necessary for his or her health. There is no reason that a person cannot ask a physician or dentist if an X-ray examination is really necessary.

Ultraviolet (UV) Radiation and Ozone

Exposure to UV radiation (part of the radiation from the sun; also called non-ionizing radiation) is greater for people who reside at higher altitudes and in areas with lots of sun. Skin cancers, such as melanoma, can result from exposure to UV radiation. Melanoma is more likely to develop in white skin than dark skin; however, the progression of melanoma in persons with dark skin is much more rapid than in white-skinned people. The use of a sunscreen may lessen the damaging effects of UV radiation during sunbathing. Some studies have reported that the combination of UV radiation and X-ray radiation is twelve times more likely to generate cancer cells than either type of radiation alone. In addition, tumor promoters present in the diet and environment also may heighten the risk of UV radiation–induced cancer formation and may be partly responsible for a fivefold increase in melanoma incidence in the Sunbelt states of the United States. We should note that chemical carcinogens that magnify the risk of X-ray-induced cancer fail to amplify the risk of UV radiation–induced cancer. The time interval between exposure to UV radiation and the formation of detectable cancer is generally more than ten years. Breathing ozone also generates free radicals, which can cause cancer.

Chemical Carcinogens

The sources of chemical carcinogens in the environment are air and water. The air may contain ozone gas, fibers (such as asbestos), and chemical particles. The burning of wood contributes to elevated levels of hydrocarbons, a powerful human carcinogen. The following chemicals are carcinogenic:

Dioxin: a by-product of herbicide and pesticide production and one of the most toxic substances to humans (exposure to only one part per billion is hazardous to human health)

Polyvinyl chloride: found in packing materials

Pesticides: found in fruits and vegetables

Polychlorinated biphenyls: present in packaging materials and in fish obtained from contaminated rivers

Diethylstilbestrol: a synthetic female hormone often fed to cattle

Polycyclic aromatic hydrocarbons, such as benzo(a)pyrene: present in air pollution

Asbestos: found in certain building materials, such as roofing and water-pipe insulation

Aflatoxin: a mold (fungus) found on peanuts and peanut butter if they are not well preserved.

Most of the chemotherapeutic agents used in the treatment of cancer also can induce cancer in human beings. It takes about ten to thirty years before a new cancer develops as the result of chemotherapy.

Biological Carcinogens

Viruses

Certain viruses, such as human T-cell leukemia viruses, SV40 (simian vacuolating virus, type 40), Epstein-Barr virus, human papillomavirus, and hepatitis C and B viruses, can be considered biological carcinogens, which have been shown to increase the risk of cancer in human beings. For example, hepatitis C and B viruses may amplify the risk of liver cancer, human papillomavirus can raise the risk of cervical cancer, and Epstein-Barr virus can magnify the risk of certain types of lymphomas (cancer of the white blood cells). These viruses have been shown to immortalize normal human cells in tissue culture and thus initiate a primary event in human carcinogenesis. The immortalized cells, after some time, sustain specific changes in certain genes, such as cellular genes, oncogenes (cancer-causing genes), or anti-oncogenes, and then become cancer cells.

Bacterial and Parasitic Infection

Human studies have shown that certain bacteria, such as *Helicobacter pylori,* raise the risk of gastric cancer, which is the most prevalent type of cancer in some developing countries. In addition, such parasites as *Opistorchis viverrini* and *Schistosoma haematobium* are considered risk factors for cholangiocarcinoma (cancer of the bile duct of the liver) and urinary bladder cancer, respectively. The removal of these infectious agents can lower the risk of these cancers. Irritation, inflammation, and induction of increased rates of division of normal cells may play a role in carcinogenesis following exposure to infectious agents. In addition, the generation of free radicals and the release of cytokines (such chemicals as tumor necrosis factor, interleukin, and prostaglandins, which can harm cells) during chronic infection may be one of the factors that magnifies the risk of cancer in infected people.

Lifestyle-Related Factors in Carcinogenesis

There are a few lifestyle-related factors that can increase the risk of some cancers. These factors include tobacco smoking or chewing, excessive consumption of alcoholic beverages or caffeine-rich beverages, excessive exposure to hyperbaric therapy, and high levels of stress.

Tobacco Smoking

It is now established that smoking tobacco products contributes to about 30 percent of all human cancers. It increases the risk not only of lung cancer but also of other cancers. Female smokers have eighty-two times the risk of lung cancer compared with nonsmoking women, whereas male smokers showed only twenty-three times the risk compared with nonsmoking men. The reasons for this marked difference in sensitivity to tobacco smoking between men and women are unknown. Chewing tobacco magnifies the risk of oral cancer. Tobacco smoking also can cause emphysema, a serious noncancerous disease with severe effects on the functioning of the lungs. In addition, smoking amplifies the risk of cardiovascular disease. There are at present more than fifty million smokers in the United States alone. Although the incidence of smoking is declining among adults, it is growing among teenagers. The public and private programs that aim to prevent smoking should be pursued vigorously. Efforts also must be made to encourage those who are addicted to tobacco smoking or chewing to quit.

What Goes On in Your Body When You Smoke?

Tobacco smoking releases cancer-causing agents into the body, enhances oxidative damage, and decreases the levels of certain antioxidants. Cigarette smoke contains a high level of nitrosamine, a potent cancer-causing agent, and nitrosating gases, which help form additional nitrosamines in the lungs. Nitrosamines are dissolved easily in water and thus can be absorbed through the mouth as well as the lungs and deposited in other organs. As a result, smoking also heightens the risk of cancer of the larynx, mouth, and esophagus and acts as a contributing factor in cancer of the urinary bladder, cervix, kidney, and pancreas.

Smoking induces several types of oxidative damage. These types include membrane damage (peroxidation), reduced levels of plasma uric acid (an important antioxidant molecule), enhanced adhesion of leukocytes (white blood cells) to the walls of blood vessels, increased aggregation of platelets (a form of blood cell), dysfunction of endothelial cells (cells that line the inner wall of blood vessels), and oxidation of plasma lipoprotein. These forms of damage can amplify the risk of heart disease.

Tobacco smoking also induces inflammatory reactions. The products of inflammatory reactions, such as free radicals and prostaglandins (a product of fatty acid, which in small amounts is essential for many cellular functions), can raise the risk of cancer. In addition, they promote oxidative damage to DNA, which can also increase the risk of cancer. Tobacco smoking lowers the levels of certain antioxidants (vitamins A and C and β-carotene), and B vitamins (cyanocobalamine and folic acid). The concentration of vitamin C declines in the breast milk of smokers, and this can add to oxidative stress in their children.

The red blood cells of smokers are more susceptible to lipid peroxidation (membrane damage) than those of nonsmokers. Supplementation with vitamin E has been reported to limit lipid peroxidation produced by free radicals. Smoking also results in folic acid deficiency, primarily affecting bronchial epithelial cells (lung cells), which become abnormal (a process called *metaplasia*). This abnormality can lead to cancer. Supplementation with 10 mg of folate and 0.5 mg of vitamin B_{12} helps curb bronchial squamous metaplasia. The data presented here suggest that persons who are in the process of quitting smoking or who are unable to quit should take a scientifically based multiple micronutrient preparation in order to lessen the oxidative damage caused by tobacco smoking.

What Is the Risk of Cancer Among Nonsmokers Who Are Exposed to Tobacco Smoke (Secondhand Smoke)?

Some human studies suggest that there is a significant increase in lung cancer risk among nonsmoking spouses of smokers. This risk is about two times higher than that found among nonsmoking couples. Smoking also can cause birth defects in the fetuses of pregnant women. The children of smoking parents (one or both partners) may have a higher risk of lung cancer. For this reason, nonsmokers should avoid surroundings with high levels of tobacco smoke. It is encouraging to note that smoking is now prohibited in many public and private places around the United States.

Heavy Drinking

About two-thirds of American adults consume alcohol, and about 17 percent of them are considered heavy drinkers. The average yearly consumption of alcohol in the United States is about 3 gallons per person. There are no data to suggest that moderate consumption of alcohol alone increases the risk of cancer, but there have been some reports that frequent drinking of wine or beer prepared in certain regions of the world (outside the United States) is associated with a higher risk of cancer of the esophagus, colon, and rectum. This risk possibly stems from impurities in the wine or beer that may be carcinogenic.

Among alcohol abusers (those who drink heavily on a constant basis), there is an increased risk of cancer of the esophagus, mouth, head and neck, lip, liver, stomach, colon, rectum, and lung. Excessive consumption of alcohol also enhances the cancer-causing effects of smoking. The combined effects of alcohol and smoking on cancer risk are about two and a half times greater than the effects associated with alcohol or smoking alone. Some researchers have suggested that intemperate consumption of alcohol may increase the risk of cancer for the following reasons:

1. Alcohol contains small amounts of cancer-causing impurities.

2. Cancer-causing substances are present in the diet and the environment, and they are also formed in the intestine. Alcohol enhances their solubility and hence the degree to which the body can absorb them. This, in turn, can heighten the risk of cancer.

3. Some agents do not act as cancer-causing substances until they are converted into an active form. Alcohol may facilitate the conversion.

4. Alcohol suppresses the body's immune defense system.

5. Alcohol may cause nutritional deficiencies, thereby raising the risk of cancer. Immoderate consumption of alcohol may lead to a deficiency in protein; vitamins A, C, and E; folic acid; thiamine (B_1); pyridoxine (B_6); and certain minerals, such as magnesium, zinc, iron, copper, and molybdenum. Deficiencies in vitamins A, C, and E may play an important role in increasing the risk of cancer induced by alcohol.

Thus, to reduce the risk of cancer of the upper intestinal tract, mouth, and lung, one should avoid excessive alcohol consumption. Those who drink moderate amounts of alcohol should not smoke at the same time and should ensure through diet and nutritional supplements that they have an adequate intake of micronutrients.

Excessive Consumption of Caffeine-Containing Beverages

Research has shown that caffeinated and decaffeinated coffee contains substances that, at high concentrations (5 to 10 cups per day), increase the frequency of radiation- and chemical-induced mutations. These results suggest that substances other than caffeine are also responsible for bringing about mutations. Similarly, certain survey-type human studies also indicate that excessive consumption of either caffeinated or decaffeinated coffee is associated with a higher risk of bladder, pancreatic, and stomach cancer, but other studies have not confirmed these results. Readily oxidized phenolic compounds that are normally present in coffee may facilitate the formation of nitrosamine from nitrite and amines in the stomach. Thus, it appears that if large amounts of nitrosamines are formed in the stomach because of a high level of coffee consumption, the risk of certain cancers, especially stomach and pancreatic cancer, may be amplified.

A recent study conducted in England reported that heavy tea consumption increases the risk of cancer of the pancreas. The cancer-causing substances in tea have not been identified. One of the factors could be caffeine. In contrast, moderate consumption of green tea or black tea has cancer-protective effects. These epidemiological human studies are not sufficient to establish a cause–effect relationship.

Caffeine has been shown to reduce the ability of cells to repair genetic damage produced spontaneously or by agents such as radiation and chemicals. It was found that normal human lymphocytes in culture exposed to low doses or irradiation (0.02 to

0.05 Gy) did not show any detectable levels of mutations. When the lymphocytes were treated with caffeine immediately after irradiation, however, mutations were evident. This study clearly indicates that caffeine can interfere with the repair of radiation-induced mutations. Therefore, too much caffeine may enhance the effect of cancer-causing substances and, in this way, act as a tumor promoter. Further laboratory and human epidemiological studies are needed to define the role of excessive consumption of caffeine in the development of human cancer.

Dietary Factors in Carcinogenesis

It has been estimated that the Western diet contributes to about 40 percent of human cancer. Human diets contain both cancer-protective and cancer-causing substances. Most of the mutagenic and carcinogenic agents present in the diet occur naturally, but other mutagens have been introduced into the diet by the use of pesticides in agricultural products. Some mutagens and carcinogens are formed during storage, cooking, and digestion, and their levels can vary markedly depending upon the type of food, storage facility, and temperature of cooking. Therefore, the relative ratio of protective versus mutagenic substances in a human diet can vary markedly from one person to another and from one day to another in the same person. In addition, fat and fiber have opposing influences in human carcinogenesis. The consumption of too much fat magnifies the risk of cancer, whereas a diet high in fiber lowers it.

Dietary Fiber and Fat

Human and animal studies suggest that a diet containing high levels of fiber may lower the risk of certain cancers, especially colon cancer. The incidence of colon cancer is virtually nil among people of northwest India (Punjabi), who eat a diet rich in roughage, cellulose, vegetables, fiber, and yogurt, compared with southern Indians, who do not eat such foods. As noted previously, the incidence of cancer in general is much lower among Seventh Day Adventists, who are vegetarians. A diet high in fiber results in regular bowel movements, which minimizes the body's contact time with cancer-causing substances normally formed in the intestinal tract. This may help limit the absorption of carcinogens and thus reduce the risk of cancer.

A high fiber intake can generate very high levels of butyric acid, owing to fermentation of fibers in the colon by bacteria. Butyric acid is a small four-carbon fatty acid that is absorbed rapidly from the colon. Butyric acid has exhibited strong anti-cancer activity against a variety of human and rodent tumor cells growing in tissue culture dishes and in certain human tumors in vivo. This may be one reason that a high-fiber diet can protect not only against intestinal cancers but also against other human cancers.

In a randomized, clinical trial, patients with familial adenomatous polyposis (precancerous lesions of the colon) who consumed an average of 22 g of total fiber, along with vitamin C (4 g per day) and α-tocopherol (400 mg per day), were found to experience a decrease in the number of polyps compared with those who received either vitamins plus low fiber (2.2 g per day) or those who received low fiber plus placebo. Reports show that only 10 percent of the U.S. population consume more than 20 g of dietary fiber daily. Excess fat acts as a tumor promoter, and, for this reason, it is recommended that a healthy person consume 20 to 25 percent of calories from fat. The average American diet contains about 40 percent of calories from fat.

Food Storage

Browning of vegetables or fruit at room temperature is an indication of the formation of mutagenic substances, such as oxidized phenolic compounds. Reduced forms of phenolic compounds are considered antioxidants. Hydrazine, a reducing agent, is often sprayed in very small amounts over salads and vegetables to prevent oxidation and thereby to keep them fresh for a longer period of time. Hydrazine can cause an allergic reaction in some people.

Cooking

Cooking at high temperatures can cause the browning of meat or vegetables. This is an indication of the formation of mutagenic substances.

What Happens When Meat Is Cooked over Charcoal?

Cooking meat over charcoal is an extremely popular practice. Studies suggest that this practice may increase the risk of cancer. If it is done in moderation and following a few simple recommendations, however, the possibility of such risk may be lowered considerably. To understand this, let us examine what happens when meat is cooked over charcoal.

As the meat cooks, fat drips down onto the hot charcoal, generating smoke that contains polycyclic aromatic hydrocarbons, such as benzo(a)pyrene, a powerful cancer-causing agent. The cooking meat is immediately exposed to and absorbs this smoke. Thus, charcoal-broiled meat contains carcinogenic substances from the smoke, whereas meat that is not charcoal-broiled does not. The amount of polycyclic aromatic hydrocarbons increases if the fat content of the meat is high and if it is cooked under conditions that expose it to high levels of fat-generated smoke. The average charcoal-broiled steak contains about 8 mcg of polycyclic aromatic hydrocarbons per kilogram of steak.

In order to minimize the levels of cancer-causing substances in charcoal-broiled meat, as much fat as possible should be removed from the meat before cooking. In addition, the meat can be placed a little farther away from the charcoal during cooking so that at least some of the fat-generated smoke will dissipate into the air before it reaches the meat. Covering the grill with aluminum foil before placing meat on it also will prevent smoke contamination. The cook and others should avoid inhaling the smoke. Alternatively, propane-powered grills can be used. In this way, people can still enjoy a barbecue without magnifying their exposure to potential cancer-causing agents.

Digestion

Mutagens and carcinogens are formed during digestion. Nitrites typically are used to preserve meat and are present in bacon, sausage, hot dogs, and cured meat. Nitrites by themselves do not cause cancer, but they can combine with amines in the stomach to form nitrosamines. Nitrosamines are among the most potent cancer-causing agents for both animals and human beings. They are soluble in water and therefore can be absorbed readily and distributed to all the tissues of the body. The presence of vitamin C or vitamin E (α-tocopherol) in the stomach may prevent the formation or lower the levels of nitrosamines.

Thus, taking vitamins C or E just before eating food containing nitrites may limit or prevent the formation of nitrosamines in the stomach. The necessary amount of either vitamin depends upon the amount of nitrites consumed. At this time, the precise amount of these vitamins needed to reduce the formation of nitrosamines has not been determined. In addition to nitrosamines, many other mutagenic substances (agents that cause genetic changes that may or may not lead to cancer) are formed in the intestinal tract. Mutations (changes in genetic material) precede cancer formation, but not all mutations lead to cancer formation.

Studies have shown that the levels of mutagenic substances in the feces are higher in persons who are meat eaters than in those who are vegetarians. The presence of higher levels of fecal mutagenic substances may increase the risk of cancer. This hypothesis is supported by the fact that the incidence of cancer among Seventh Day Adventists, who are vegetarians, is much lower than among people who eat meat. It has been reported that taking vitamin C or vitamin E reduces the levels of mutagenic substances in the feces of meat eaters. Furthermore, reports indicate that taking both vitamins is more effective than taking either individually. Therefore, an appropriate preparation of multiple antioxidants with B vitamins and suitable minerals taken before meals may curb the formation of mutagenic and carcinogenic agents in the gastrointestinal tract.

Nutrients That May Increase the Risk of Cancer
Excess Total Fat

Both human studies and animal experiments suggest that increasing the total fat intake raises the risk of certain cancers, particularly breast, colon, prostate, and possibly other cancers. Conversely, lowering fat intake lessens the risk of these cancers. High levels of fat, therefore, act as a tumor promoter. Data from animal studies suggest that when total fat intake is low, polyunsaturated fats are more likely than saturated fats to promote cancer, but the relevance of this observation for human beings is not clear at this time. In addition, specific components of fat responsible for enhanced carcinogenesis have not been identified, though some studies indicate that excess cholesterol consumption may increase the risk of cancer. Extensive human studies are needed to define the role of too much cholesterol in carcinogenesis.

There is no exact explanation for the effects of a high-fat diet on cancer risk, but some laboratory experiments have reported that the production of prostaglandin E_2 (PGE_2), a chemical that is produced by the body, is greatly increased in animals that are fed a high-fat diet. High levels of PGE_2 have been shown to impair the body's immune defense system. Therefore, the amplified risk of cancer brought about by a high-fat diet may be due to the suppression of the body's defense system against cancer. High doses of vitamin E have been reported to diminish the production of PGE_2, and, consequently, high doses of vitamin E may block some of the harmful effects of excessive fat consumption. This does not mean that one should continue eating a high-fat diet and take large amounts of vitamin E, since a high-fat diet may also heighten the risk of heart attack. The relationship between diet and lifestyle and cancer risk is listed in Table 2.

A high-fat diet can raise the levels of circulating estrogen in females, and estrogen is known to act as a tumor promoter. The presence in the human body of large amounts of bile acids and fatty acids from a diet rich in fat may promote colon cancer, because these substances encourage the proliferation of cells in the colon. Increased cell proliferation makes colon cells more sensitive to cancer formation. Dietary calcium inhibits this action of bile acids and fatty acids by making them insoluble and rendering them unavailable for absorption.

Excess Protein

Limited laboratory data and human studies suggest that an immoderate intake of protein may be associated with a higher risk of cancer of the breast, endometrium, prostate, colon, rectum, pancreas, and kidney. A lower protein intake seems to reduce the risk of cancer. Although animal studies suggest that protein has a specific role in animal carcinogenesis, human studies are not persuasive. Since the Western diet contains significant amounts of meat, which is a rich source of both protein and fat, it is difficult at this time to determine the independent role of protein in human carcinogenesis. The fact that animal experiments show that a high protein intake increases the incidence of chemically induced tumors, however, indicates that proteins may have a similar role in human cancer. Additional studies are needed to substantiate this particular point.

Table 2 — Probable Causative Agent of Various Types of Cancer

Causative Agent	Type of Cancer
Excess fat	Prostate, breast, stomach, colon, rectum, pancreas, and ovary
Excess protein	Breast, endometrium, prostate, colon, rectum, pancreas, kidney
Excess total calorie intake	Most cancers
Excess alcohol	Esophagus, mouth, head and neck, lip, stomach, liver, colon, rectum
Smoking	Lung, larynx, mouth, esophagus
Excess alcohol plus smoking	Mouth, larynx, esophagus, lung
Excess coffee or alcohol, smoking	Pancreas, lung, liver, mouth, larynx, esophagus
Excess coffee, tea	Bladder, pancreas, stomach
Excess saccharine	Bladder
Cadmium from diet, smoking	Kidney
Excess zinc	All cancers, especially breast and stomach
Iron deficiency	Stomach and esophagus
Iodine deficiency	Thyroid
Excess smoked meat or fish, charcoal-broiled meat, pickled products	Stomach
Certain viruses	Liver, certain blood cancers

Excess Total Calories and Carbohydrates
There are limited studies that suggest that increased total caloric intake may increase the risk of cancer, but the data on both animals and human beings are sparse and indirect. Further studies are needed to answer this question. There are no scientific data to suggest that an excessive intake of carbohydrates is directly related to the risk of cancer in animals or human beings. However, excessive consumption of carbohydrates may increase total caloric intake. Additional studies are needed to define the role of carbohydrates in human carcinogenesis.

Concluding Remarks

Many human cancers are associated with environmental, dietary, and lifestyle-related factors. Therefore, the risk of many cancers can be modified with changes in these factors. Nonetheless, a single person cannot control the levels of carcinogens present in the environment. It requires government regulation, which is not easily accomplished. We can control our diet and lifestyle-related factors, however. The incidence of human cancer can be reduced significantly with such modifications.

5 Cancer Prevention Studies and Recommendations

Despite extensive research on the role of diet, antioxidants, and lifestyle-related factors in the prevention of cancer, the public and health professionals remain confused on this issue owing to contradictory results on the use of supplemental micronutrients (antioxidants, B vitamins, and appropriate minerals) published in scientific journals. Contradictory results stem from the fact that human studies are often performed without scientific rationale with respect to dose, type, chemical form, and number of appropriate antioxidants. In addition, modifications in diet and lifestyle are often overlooked while investigating the role of antioxidants in cancer prevention. Many published studies support the idea that a moderate supplement of multiple antioxidants, B vitamins, and appropriate minerals, as well as modifications in diet and lifestyle, are equally important for a maximal effect on cancer prevention. Cancer prevention studies have been performed on three experimental models: cell culture models, animal models, and human models.

Experimental Models of Cancer Prevention

Cell Culture Model

In this model, normal cells are grown in tissue culture dishes of varying sizes (30 to 100 centimeters in diameter) containing solutions of nutrients that are necessary for cell growth. This cell culture model is also referred to as an *in vitro model.* This term is misleading, because "in vitro" often refers to test tube studies in which experiments are performed with broken cell preparations, whereas in the cell culture model, studies are performed on intact cells. In cancer prevention studies, one group of dishes containing cells is pretreated with specific antioxidants before being exposed to carcinogens. Antioxidants are allowed to remain in the dishes for the entire period of observation. Another group of dishes with cells is treated with the carcinogen alone for the same length of time. These two groups of cells are allowed to grow for a specified period of time. Generally, within 6 to 12 weeks of treatment with a carcinogen, a small percentage of normal cells become cancer cells. The presence of antioxidants markedly reduces the number of cells that become cancerous.

The cell culture model is a very good experimental system for identifying potential cancer-causing agents and cancer-protective substances. In addition, it allows one to determine the efficacy of cancer-causing or cancer-protective agents within a short time interval. This model also permits one to study the direct effect of experimental agents without the influence of variations in absorption, metabolism, and excretion, which are commonly found in animal or human models. Furthermore, one can define the genetic changes responsible for cancer formation or cancer protection. These genetic studies on cancer cannot be undertaken using animal or human models with any accuracy. Thus, the cell culture model is considered both cost- and time-effective, but the results obtained from cell culture studies cannot be extrapolated readily to animals or humans with respect to dose, toxicity, or level of efficacy. Certain types of studies, such as those assessing the effect of large amounts of fiber in cancer prevention, cannot be performed with this model, because the protective role of fiber involves the gastrointestinal tract. In addition, the effects of compounds requiring metabolic activation by liver enzymes for their biological activity cannot be evaluated in a standard cell culture model.

Many cell culture studies have shown consistently that some individual antioxidants at high doses can lessen the incidence of chemical- or radiation-induced cancer. Low doses of certain antioxidants can stimulate the growth of specific cancer cells. This finding is significant, since some of the human cancer prevention trials focusing on a single nutrient have utilized low doses and are conducted among high-risk groups, who, in some cases, may have undetectable precancerous or cancerous cells. As expected from the cell culture studies, such human studies show an increased incidence of certain types of cancer following supplementation with a low-dose single antioxidant.

Animal Model

Primarily rodents (rats, mice, and hamsters) are used as animal models in cancer prevention studies. A group of animals is treated with a carcinogen subcutaneously (under the skin) or intraperitoneally (into the abdominal cavity). Another group of animals is given a carcinogen in the same manner, but they also receive individual antioxidants through local application to the skin site where the chemical carcinogen is applied, before treatment with the carcinogen or at various times after treatment with the carcinogen. It takes about a year for a tumor to appear in a group of animals receiving a carcinogen alone. The incidence rates of tumors are compared for the two groups of animals.

A genetically engineered animal, called a transgenic mouse, has been developed for use in cancer studies. A mutated oncogene is introduced into an egg and then implanted into the uterus of the female mouse. All animals born by this method express the mutated oncogene at birth, resulting in a high incidence of various types of cancer during their adult life. This model also is being used in cancer prevention studies.

Numerous animal studies have confirmed the cancer-preventive role of antioxidants and a high-fiber, low-fat diet and the cancer-enhancing role of excess fat, carbohydrate, protein, and calories. Some studies also have confirmed that individual antioxidants at certain doses can enhance chemical-induced cancer. Thus, animal studies corroborate the results of cell studies, which suggest that single specific antioxidants at high doses can decrease cancer incidence but at low doses can enhance the incidence of certain cancers among high-risk populations.

Human Model

Two distinct models are used to evaluate the role of micronutrients, diet, and lifestyle on the incidence of human cancer: the epidemiological study and the intervention trial. The epidemiological study is based primarily on the determination of levels of micronutrients, type of diet, and lifestyles based on the answers of participants to questionnaires and the correlation of these results with the incidence of cancer. They use two experimental designs, a retrospective case-control study and a prospective case-control study.

Epidemiologic Studies

The design of a retrospective case-control study involves an analysis of the history of dietary intake in cancer patients compared with that in age- and sex-matched healthy people. From this comparison, the correlation of dietary factors and incidence of cancer is estimated. The design of a prospective case-control study entails an analysis of dietary intake from diet records among selected populations and correlation of the levels of micronutrients, type of diet, and lifestyle with the incidence of cancer among these groups.

From the dietary intake data obtained through questionnaires, measures of the amounts of antioxidants (such as vitamins A, C, and E and β-carotene) and the levels of fat and fiber are generated using appropriate nutrition-related computer software. Occasionally, the blood levels of these nutrients are measured and correlated with the incidence of cancer. Using the experimental designs cited earlier, most studies have reported that a diet rich in antioxidants, low in fat, and high in fiber is associated with a lower risk of human cancers. Some studies, however, have found no such relationship. Others have reported that when the risk of cancer is correlated with the levels of individual antioxidants, the association with reduced cancer incidence is weak or nonexistent or even reversed.

Epidemiological and experimental studies suggest that daily consumption of four or more cups of green tea has cancer-protective value. The main protective components of green tea are epigallocatchin and other phenols, which are antioxidants. They also inhibit the growth of cancer cells.

There have been no studies on cancer risk in which the combined effect of a diet rich in antioxidants, low in fat, and high in fiber was evaluated. This is very important, because human diets contain agents that produce opposite effects on cancer risk. For example, a diet rich in antioxidants, high in fiber, and low in fat is cancer protective, whereas a diet rich in fat, meat, and nitrites and low in antioxidants and fiber may increase the risk of cancer.

Dietary factors also can influence the metabolism of mutagens and carcinogens.

Under the best experimental conditions, human epidemiological studies can only suggest an association between a nutrient and cancer risk. Often, such data are interpreted in the lay press as asserting a cause-and-effect relationship between levels of micronutrients and cancer risk, which is misleading. Any question raised by an epidemiological study must be tested by an intervention trial among high-risk groups. Only when the findings are confirmed in an intervention trial can epidemiological data be considered valid in establishing cause and effect between nutrients and cancer incidence.

Intervention Trials

This type of study is performed among high-risk populations using one or more micronutrients. One group receives antioxidants, and another group receives a placebo (a sugar pill with no antioxidants). To evaluate the efficacy of treatment, the incidence of cancer and/or markers of cancer is determined. Results of several published intervention trials have been contradictory, owing to the fact that these studies have failed to consider biologic rationales developed from studies on cell culture, animal models, and human epidemiological investigations. Some studies have used a low-dose single nutrient; others have used one or more nutrients, including antioxidants, without addressing the need for modification in the diet and lifestyle. It is essential to administer appropriate doses of nutrients, including several antioxidants, together with modifications in diet and lifestyle in any intervention trial, for maximal effect on cancer prevention.

Effects of Antioxidants: Relevance to Cancer Prevention

Antioxidants perform several biological functions that are pertinent to cancer prevention. Some of these effects are described here.

Antioxidants as Scavengers of Free Radicals

One of the well-established mechanisms of action of antioxidants, such as vitamins A, C, and E, and carotenoids, such as β-carotene, lutein, and lycopene, involves protecting cells from free radical damage. In addition, other constituents of plant food, such as phenolic compounds, exhibit antioxidant properties. Free radicals are generated as a natural consequence of oxidative metabolism. These free radicals are highly reactive and cause damage to biological molecules, such as protein, lipid, membranes, DNA (a cell's genetic material), and RNA (which carries the genetic code for making protein). Free radicals have been implicated as playing a key role in human carcinogenesis, and it would seem to follow that antioxidant supplements should have cancer-protective value. Not all antioxidants have the same efficacy in removing different types of free radicals within varying cellular environments, however.

For example, β-carotene acts as a more efficient quencher of oxygen-free radicals compared with other antioxidants. It is an especially effective antioxidant under reduced oxygen pressure. Alpha-tocopheryl succinate (α-TS), a form of vitamin E, is more effective than α-tocopherol. Furthermore, vitamin C is a potent antioxidant in a water environment, whereas vitamin A, β-carotene, and vitamin E work well in a lipid environment. These observations suggest that a mixture of antioxidants may be more efficacious than individual antioxidants in cancer prevention, because they can impart optimal protection against free-radical damage throughout the organism.

Prevention of the Formation of Potential Carcinogens in the Gut

Carcinogenic and mutagenic agents are formed during storage, digestion, and metabolism of food, and antioxidants can limit the formation of these agents. For example, the consumption of nitrite-rich food (such as bacon, sausage, and cured meat) can form nitrosamines in the stomach at an acid pH by the combination of nitrites and secondary amines. The presence of vitamin C or vitamin E averts this reaction in the human gastrointestinal tract, which may lower the risk of cancer among those who consume nitrite-rich foods. Diets rich in meat increase the levels of mutagenic substances in the feces compared with vegetarian diets. Daily intake of vitamin C or vitamin E decreases the amount of mutagenic substances in the feces; the combination of vitamin C and vitamin E is more effective than either antioxidant alone. Human studies suggest that certain antioxidants can prevent the formation of carcinogens and mutagens in the gastrointestinal tract.

Prevention of the Conversion of Inactive to Active Carcinogens in the Liver

Some indirect carcinogens, such as nitrosamine and benzo(a)pyrene, are not carcinogenic until they are converted into active forms in the liver by oxidation reactions. High levels of antioxidants in the liver may forestall this reaction and thereby reduce the risk of cancer among those who are absorbing high levels of indirect carcinogens. These inactive carcinogens are then excreted in the urine.

Induction of Cell Differentiation, Growth Inhibition, or Both in Cancer Cells in Culture

Certain antioxidants can induce cell differentiation (converting cancer cells to cells that are more normal), growth inhibition of cancer cells, or both, depending upon the dose and type of antioxidants and the type of tumor cell. For example, individual retinoids (vitamin A) have been found to induce differentiation and growth inhibition in several human and rodent tumor cell types. Alpha-tocopheryl succinate also has brought about cell differentiation and growth inhibition in several human and rodent tumor cells in culture, whereas α-tocopherol and α-tocopheryl acetate were inactive. This finding suggests that α-TS is the most active form of vitamin E. Beta-carotene and vitamin C also inhibit the growth of some cancer cells in culture.

Stimulation of the Growth of Certain Cancer Cells

In contrast to higher doses, low doses of individual antioxidants can stimulate the growth of some cancer cells in culture. For example, vitamin C alone encourages the growth of human leukemia cells and human parotid carcinoma cells. Beta-carotene alone also can incite the growth of human melanoma cells in culture. The same doses of antioxidants do not encourage the growth of other types of tumor cells. If the same low doses are used in a mixture of antioxidants, they never stimulate the growth of any cancer cell. Thus, the use of single antioxidants at low doses in cancer prevention trials may be ineffective or even harmful among high-risk populations in which some people may already have precancerous or cancerous lesions that are too small to be detected clinically.

Induction of Growth Inhibition in Some Tumor Cells But Not in Normal Cells in Living Organisms

As mentioned earlier, vitamin C, α-TS, β-carotene, and retinoids at high doses inhibited the growth of some tumor cells in rodents and humans. These antioxidants have no growth-inhibitory effects on normal cells, however. This lack of effect may be related in part to the difference in the uptake of antioxidants. Tumor cells can accumulate higher amounts of these antioxidants than normal cells. The high intracellular levels of antioxidants in tumor cells can lead to cell death, differentiation, or growth inhibition, depending on the concentration of antioxidants, types of antioxidants, and types of cancer cells. In some cases, normal and cancer cells may accumulate similar levels of antioxidants; however, tumor cells become more sensitive to antioxidants than normal cells.

Apoptosis in Cancer Cells But Not in Normal Cells

Apoptosis refers to the process of cell death in which cells show signs of fragmented nuclear DNA. Several studies have investigated the role of antioxidants in regulating apoptotic events in both normal and cancer cells in culture. These studies have shown that certain antioxidants can induce apoptosis in tumor cells but not in normal cells. They also protect normal cells against chemical-induced apoptosis.

Interactions Between Antioxidants

Although extensive studies have been undertaken to investigate the effects of individual antioxidants on the growth and differentiation of tumor cells in culture and in living organisms, very few studies have been carried out to evaluate the effects of several antioxidants on the growth of tumor cells. Recent studies show that several antioxidants, even at low doses, inhibit the growth of cancer cells. In general, antioxidants taken together are more effective in suppressing the growth of tumor cells in culture than single antioxidants. In designing any human intervention trial among high-risk groups, the importance of synergism between antioxidants must be considered.

Interaction Between Antioxidants and Other Physiologic Substances

Antioxidants not only have a direct effect on tumor cells, individually or in combination, they also modify the effect of some physiologic agents on cell differentiation and growth inhibition. For example, α-TS and β-carotene enhance the effect of adenosine 3',5'-cyclic monophosphate (cAMP), a substance present in all human cells, on the differentiation of the cells of neuroblastoma (a childhood cancer of embryonic nerve cells) in culture. As we have said, differentiation is the process that converts cancer cells to normal cells. Alpha-tocopheryl succinate also increases the extent of cAMP-induced differentiation in melanoma cells in culture. Vitamin C, α-TS, β-carotene, and retinoids magnify the growth-inhibitory effects of interferon alpha-2b (an immune stimulant compound) on human melanoma cells in culture. Retinoids enhance the growth-inhibitory effects of interferon alpha-2a on human cervical squamous cell carcinoma in vivo. Alpha-tocopheryl succinate and vitamin C also amplify the growth-inhibitory effect of sodium butyrate, a four-carbon fatty acid with strong anticancer activity on cancer cells in culture and in living organisms. These results highlight a novel function of antioxidants—the enhancement of the effect of other physiological substances in the body.

Reduction of the Action of Prostaglandin E$_1$

High levels of prostaglandins (PGs) act as tumor promoters for some types of cancer. A high-fat diet raises the level of PGs in animals and likewise may increase the incidence of chemical-induced cancer. Anti-inflammatory drugs, such as aspirin and indomethacin, which limit the production of PGs, lower the risk of chemical-induced cancer in animals. These results suggest that excessive levels of PGs may increase the incidence of chemical-induced cancer. Alpha-tocopheryl succinate inhibits the action of PGs in mammalian cells in culture. A combination of vitamin C and vitamin E inhibits PGE_2 synthesis and release. These results suggest that a combination of nonsteroidal anti-inflammatory drugs and several antioxidants may lessen the risk of PG-mediated carcinogenesis more effectively than individual agents alone.

Reduction of the Incidence of Mutations

Random mutations due to chromosomal aberrations or gene defects alone are not sufficient to cause cancer, but they are considered one of the risk factors for cancer formation. Vitamins C and E and β-carotene decrease chromosomal damage produced by ionizing radiation and chemical carcinogens. Supplementation with high doses of antioxidants curbs oxygen free radical–induced damage to DNA in human lymphocytes. These antioxidants must be present at high levels in the cells before their exposure to carcinogens. High-dose antioxidants can prevent mutations due to chromosomal damage and gene changes and thus can reduce the risk of cancer.

Regulation of Gene Expression in Cancer Cells

Many studies now indicate that certain antioxidants can regulate the expression of cellular genes and oncogenes in tumor cells in culture. Some effects of antioxidants on cell differentiation and growth inhibition in tumor cells may be related to alterations in gene expression. Tables 3 and 4 list the changes in gene expression in tumor cells in culture; NA=not available.

Table 3 — Effect of δ-Alpha-Tocopheryl Succinate or Aqueous Vitamin E on Gene Expression and/or Activity in Tumor Cells

Reduced Gene Expression and/or Activity	Increased Gene Expression and/or Activity
Mutated p21	Normal p21
Mutated p53	Normal p53
c-*myc*	TGF-β
N-*myc*	Protein kinase A activity
H-*ras*	NA
VEGF	NA
Protein kinase C activity	NA

p21 and p53 are tumor-suppressor genes; c-*myc*, N-*myc*, and H-*ras* are oncogenes. VEGF (vascular endothelial growth factor) and TGF-β (transforming growth factor β) are cellular genes. The levels of mRNA of these genes represent expression. Protein kinase C was expressed as enzyme activity.

Table 4 — Effect of Retinoids and Beta-Carotene on Gene Expression and/or Activity in Tumor Cells

Reduced Gene Expression and/or Activity	Increased Gene Expression and/or Activity
Mutated p53	Normal p53
c-*myc*	c-*fos*
H-*ras*	c-*jun*
c-*neu*	HSP70
c-*erb*-β2	HSP90
Phosphotyrosine kinase activity	Cyclin A and D and their kinases activities
NA	MAP kinase

p53 is a tumor-suppressor gene; c-*myc*, H-*ras*, c-*neu*, and c-*erb*-β2 are oncogenes, whereas c-*fos*, c-*jun*, HSP (heat-shock protein) 70 and HSP90, and cyclin A and D are cellular genes. Phosphotyrosine kinase and MAP kinase are enzymes.

These changes in gene expression in tumor cells are responsible for the effect of antioxidants on cell differentiation and growth inhibition. The p53 gene is considered to be a tumor-suppressor gene, or an anti-oncogene. A mutation in p53 makes this gene ineffective and thus heightens the risk of cancer. It is important to note that antioxidants can decrease the expression of the mutated form of p53, whereas they enhance the expression of wild-type (normal) p53.

Beta-carotene strengthens the expression of the connexin gene, which makes a gap junction protein that is responsible for maintaining the link between two normal cells. Cancer cells are found to have diminished activity of the connexin gene. Retinoids and other antioxidants do not produce this effect of β-carotene, suggesting that it may be unique to β-carotene. The high level of expression of the connexin gene may be one of the explanations of β-carotene-induced cancer prevention in mammalian cells in culture. Studies on the role of antioxidants in gene regulation are emerging, and more investigations should be undertaken to elucidate the regulation of gene activity by antioxidants at the levels of transcription and translation of genes. Results of studies on gene alteration clearly indicate that antioxidants can induce cell differentiation and growth inhibition in several ways, including alterations in the expression of oncogenes and other cellular genes.

Stimulation of the Host's Immune System

Although the host's immune system may not play a direct part in cellular transformation, it could have an important role in rejecting newly transformed cells. The optimally functioning immune system can recognize transformed cells and kill them. A weak immune system may allow the establishment of newly transformed cells and eventual conversion to malignant cells. Vitamins A, C, and E and β-carotene at high doses enhance immune function.

Low-dose daily supplementation with antioxidants, such as vitamin C (120 mg), β-carotene (6 mg), vitamin E (15 mg), zinc (20 mg), and selenium (100 mcg), improve antioxidant defense system after 6 months of supplementation. Antioxidant-induced cancer prevention in a living organism may be due in part to the stimulation of the host's immune system.

The studies discussed here show that the effects of antioxidants at the cellular level are very complex and that some are directly relevant to cancer prevention. Therefore, the cancer-preventive action of antioxidants has a sound basis in laboratory experiments. The cancer-preventive actions of β-carotene, selenium, and vitamins A, C, and E are listed in Table 5.

Table 5 — Summary of the Actions of Antioxidants and Selenium in Cancer Prevention

Nutrients	Preventive Action
Vitamin C and vitamin E (α-tocopherol)	Block the formation of cancer-causing agents
Most antioxidants	Block the conversion of some cancer-causing agents to active forms
Beta-carotene, vitamin A (retinol and retinoic acid), vitamin C, vitamin E (α-tocopherol, α-TS), and selenium	Block the action of tumor-causing agents (initiators and promoters)
Beta-carotene; vitamins A, C, and E	Reverse newly formed cancer cells back to normal cells
Beta-carotene; vitamins A, C, E; and selenium	Kill newly formed cancer cells in the body by stimulating the body's immune defense system

Studies on Diet and Cancer Incidence in Different Countries

The relationship of diet and lifestyle to cancer has been observed in many parts of the world. Some examples are given here.

Japan

A high incidence of stomach cancer has been associated with the consumption of spices and pickled food. The rate of stomach cancer is markedly lower among Japanese immigrants who adopt Western food habits; however, the incidence of stomach cancer remains high among Japanese immigrants in the United States who continue to follow Japanese dietary habits. The incidence of breast cancer is low among Japanese women compared with American or European women. This finding has been attributed to a difference in the fat content of the diet, which also accounts for a difference in the level of circulating blood levels of estrogen. Japanese women, who often eat a low-fat diet, have lower levels of blood estrogen than women in the United States, who usually eat a diet higher in fat. Higher levels of estrogen are known to increase the risk of breast cancer.

Chile

The high incidence of stomach cancer in Chile appears to be associated with the consumption of food and drinking water that contain relatively high levels of nitrate, a chemical that combines with other chemicals (amines) in the stomach to form nitrosamine, a potent cancer-causing substance. The high rate of bacterial infection also contributes to an increased rate of occurrence of gastric cancer.

Iceland

The incidence of stomach cancer among Icelanders who consume large quantities of smoked fish and meat is much higher than among those who eat such food in smaller amounts. Smoked fish contains high levels of hydrocarbons (cancer-causing agents) that are formed during smoking.

India

The high rate of oral cancer in India is associated with chewing betel nuts, which contain several cancer-causing agents. The habit of holding dry tobacco leaves between the lip and gum is associated with an increased incidence of lip cancer. This form of cancer is not unique to India but is common to all regions where people chew tobacco. Colon cancer is virtually absent among the Punjabi people in northwest India, who eat a diet rich in cellulose, vegetables, fiber, and yogurt.

United States

The incidence of stomach cancer has declined recently because of changing dietary habits. The rates of colon and rectal cancer among Seventh Day Adventists, who eat a vegetarian diet, is much lower than among persons who eat meat. In addition, Mormons, who do not smoke, drink alcohol, or consume excess caffeine, have a lower incidence of colon and rectal cancer. The consumption of a diet low in fiber and high in fat contributes to the heightened incidence of various cancers, including breast, colon, and prostate cancer.

China

In one province of China, there is a high rate of occurrence of esophageal cancer. This appears to be related to the fact that the selenium content of the soil is very low. The people of this region eat mostly pickled food and only small quantities of fruits and vegetables. From these regional studies, it is clear that diet- and lifestyle-related factors play an important role in determining the risk of cancer.

Intervention Trials with Antioxidants Among High-Risk Populations

The failure of intervention studies to consider scientific rationales developed by laboratory and human epidemiological studies has led to the reporting of contradictory results. Some of the published studies are summarized here. The data presented in Table 6 show that the oral administration of more than one nutrient, as well as antioxidants at high doses and bacille Calmette-Guérin (BCG) vaccine, lowers the rate of recurrence of human bladder cancer by 40 percent in five years compared with a daily multiple antioxidant supplement with the RDA value of each nutrient. BCG vaccine is known to act as an immune stimulant. This is an impressive and promising result, even though no diet or lifestyle modifications were addressed and the impact of dietary fat and fiber was not evaluated.

Table 6 — Effect of High-Dose Multiple Antioxidants on the Recurrence of Human Bladder Cancer

Micronutrients per Day	Outcome
Vitamin A, 40,000 IU Vitamin C, 2,000 mg Vitamin E, 400 IU Vitamin B_6, 100 mg A multiple vitamin containing RDA value of each nutrient BCG vaccine	40% of bladder cancers recurred
A multiple vitamin containing RDA value of each nutrient	80% of bladder cancers recurred

Another study, which was performed in a rural hospital in Italy, showed that daily oral consumption of a mixture of high-dose multiple antioxidants reduced the recurrence of colon polyps (adenomas) by 30 percent. A daily intake of a large amount of fiber also minimized the recurrence of colon polyps by 21 percent (Table 7). It remains to be established whether a combination of several high-dose antioxidants with a high-fiber diet would produce more impressive results. Changes in lifestyle were not addressed in this study. Such changes may have enhanced the efficacy of this micronutrient regimen.

Table 7 — Effect of Several High-Dose Antioxidants on the Recurrence of Colorectal Adenoma among Italians

Micronutrients per Day	Outcome
Vitamin A, 3,000 IU Vitamin C, 1,000 mg Vitamin E, 70 mg	30% reduction in recurrence
Lactulose, 20 g	21% reduction in recurrence

In contrast to this study, a U.S. investigation reported no beneficial effects of high-dose combination antioxidants on the recurrence of colon polyps. The U.S. study utilized the following antioxidants: synthetic β-carotene, 25 mg per day; vitamin C, 1,000 mg per day; and vitamin E, 400 mg per day.

These two intervention trials, which examined the effects of several high-dose antioxidants on the reduction of the recurrence of colon polyps, are difficult to compare. The Italian study used vitamin A, whereas the U.S. study used synthetic β-carotene. Synthetic β-carotene has been found to be inactive in some biological systems. It has been reported that some preparations of synthetic β-carotene have no active β-carotene. The U.S. study did not measure the purity of its synthetic β-carotene. For an optimal effect, both natural β-carotene and vitamin A should have been used. A relatively inactive form of vitamin E (synthetic α-tocopherol) was used in the U.S. study. No modifications in diet or lifestyle were recommended in either study. It would be reasonable to assume that patients in the rural Italian hospital had a lower-fat diet compared with the patients in the United States.

The value of diet in cancer prevention trials is underscored by another U.S. study, which reported that vitamin C (4 g per day) and vitamin E (400 mg per day) in combination with a high-fiber diet of more than 12 g per day for a period of four years reduced the recurrence of colon polyps more than the same dose of antioxidants without large amounts of fiber. This study emphasizes the importance of dietary fiber in intervention trials using several antioxidants. A low fat intake was not recommended in this study. Such a diet may have further lessened the recurrence of colon polyps. Another randomized trial, using 400 mg of vitamin C and 400 mg of synthetic vitamin E (dl-α-tocopherol), failed to limit the recurrence of colon polyps. No diet or lifestyle modifications were recommended in this study. This study did not follow scientific rationale with respect to dose, type, and chemical form of antioxidants; number of antioxidants; or diet and lifestyle. In another study, multiple vitamins, vitamin E, and calcium supplements were found to be associated with a lower rate of recurrence of adenoma in patients with a history of colon cancer.

A joint U.S. and Chinese study found that high-dose (two to three times the RDA) multiple micronutrients (β-carotene, vitamin E, and selenium) reduced mortality rates by 10 percent and cancer incidence by 13 percent in a high-risk population. This study also made no suggestion concerning diet or lifestyle modifications, but it can be assumed that the Chinese in rural areas consume less fat and fewer calories than Americans. Another finding of the study was that long-term consumption of 4 cups or more of green tea per day is associated with lower recurrence rates of stages I and II breast cancer.

In contrast to the reported beneficial results of high-dose combination antioxidants in some studies, other trials using low doses of individual antioxidants reported detrimental effects among high-risk populations. For example, one study suggested that synthetic β-carotene at a dose of 20 mg per day may increase the incidence of lung cancer by 17 percent among men who smoke heavily. Supplementation with α-tocopherol at a dose of 50 mg per day reduced the rate of prostate and colorectal cancers but enhanced the incidence of stomach cancer. No modifications in diet or lifestyle were recommended in any of these studies. The studies are consistent, however, in terms of laboratory data, which suggest that small doses of individual antioxidants can stimulate the growth of some cancer cells and have no effect or beneficial effects on some other cancer cells.

This concept is supported by another intervention trial in which selenium was given daily at a dose of 200 mcg. No modifications in diet or lifestyle were recommended in this study. The consumption of this dose of selenium did not have any significant effect on the incidence of skin cancer, but it did lower the rate of prostate cancer. There was a slight increase in the incidence of endometrial cancer in this group, though it was not considered statistically significant.

Thus, the use of low doses of single micronutrients in any cancer prevention trial among a high-risk population has no scientific merit. In fact, such trials could be harmful in the case of some cancers. In contrast to the observations about the effects of low doses of β-carotene taken by persons at high risk of cancer, such doses of β-carotene did not produce these effects among normal, healthy people.

In some cases, very high doses of individual antioxidants could have beneficial effects in terms of lowering the risk of some types of cancer in high-risk populations, but such doses could also be toxic. For example, vitamin A supplementation at a dose of 300,000 IU per day for 12 months effected an 11 percent reduction in the recurrence rate of primary non–small cell lung carcinoma, but this high dose of vitamin A cannot be taken over a long period of time owing to its toxicity. High doses of β-carotene, retinoids, and *dl*-β-tocopherol alone or in combination cause varying degrees of regression of oral leukoplakia, a precancerous lesion of oral cancer. A partial list of intervention trails is given in Table 8.

Table 8 — A Partial List of Intervention Trials

Patient Group	Randomized Agent	Investigator/Institution
Nonfamilial polyps	High vs. low wheat Wheat bran fiber	D. Alberts, U. of Arizona, Tucson, AZ
Nonfamilial polyps	Aspirin vs. placebo	J. Baron, Dartmouth, Hanover, NH
Nonfamilial polyps	Low fat/5 to 8 servings of fruits and vegetables vs. standard diet	A. Schatzkin, National Cancer Institute, Bethesda, MD
Women at increased risk of breast cancer	Low-fat diet	W. Insull, Baylor College of Medicine, Houston, TX
Breast cancer	4-hydroxyphenyl Retinamide	U. Veronesi, Istituto Nazionale, Milan, Italy
Cervical dysplasia	Trans-retinoic acid	E. A. Surwit, U. of Arizona, Tucson, AZ
General population from high-risk area	Multiple vitamins, β-carotene	P. Taylor, NCI, Chinese Academy of Medical Science, Beijing, China

Table 8 — A Partial List of Intervention Trials, continued

Patient Group	Randomized Agent	Investigator/Institution
Tin miners in China (lung cancer)	Beta-carotene, retinal vitamin E, selenium	A. Schatzkin, National Cancer Institute, Bethesda, MD
Basal cell carcinoma/ actinic keratoses	Retinol	T. Moon, U. of Arizona, Tucson, AZ
Basal cell carcinoma/ (male military and Veterans Affairs hospital patients)	13-cis-retinoic acid	J. Tangrea, National Cancer Institute, Bethesda, MD
Basal cell carcinoma/ squamous cell carcinoma	Retinol, 13-cis-retinoic acid	F. Meyskens, University of California Cancer Center, Irvine, CA

Conclusions Based on Laboratory, Epidemiological, and Intervention Studies

The conclusions drawn from our survey of initial laboratory, epidemiological, and intervention studies on antioxidant supplements, diet, and lifestyle modifications are summarized here.

1. High doses of such individual antioxidants as retinoids, vitamin C, vitamin E, and β-carotene are needed to reduce the risk of chemical- and radiation-induced cancers in animals and in normal cells in culture. Laboratory animals or normal cells exposed to carcinogens are analogous to human populations with a high risk of cancer (e.g., smokers). Therefore, cancer prevention trials among high-risk groups of people should use high doses of individual antioxidants if the efficacy of a single micronutrient is to

be evaluated. High doses of certain antioxidants can be toxic, however, especially if consumed over a long period of time. For this reason, high doses of individual antioxidants cannot be considered an effective strategy for cancer prevention.

2. Human epidemiological studies in general have shown that diets rich in antioxidants are associated with a lower risk of cancer. When individual dietary antioxidant intake is correlated with cancer risk, the level of decline in cancer incidence diminishes, becomes negligible, or even increases. This suggests that cancer prevention trials must use supplements containing several antioxidants rather than single antioxidants.

3. The dose of each antioxidant in a multiple micronutrient preparation would depend upon the risk status of the human population. Cancer prevention protocols can be separately developed for high-risk and normal-risk groups. High-risk groups include heavy tobacco smokers, asbestos workers, uranium miners, cancer patients in remission after conventional therapy, people with the risk of recurrence of premalignant lesions, and people with familial risk factors. Higher doses of multiple antioxidants are needed for high-risk populations than for the normal population.

4. Both laboratory and human epidemiological studies have indicated that a high-fiber diet lowers the risk of cancer, whereas a high-fat diet amplifies the risk. Human diets contain ingredients that have opposing influences on cancer incidence. To obtain maximal reduction in cancer incidence, a cancer prevention protocol that uses multiple antioxidants must also include suggestions for diet modification with respect to low fat and high fiber.

5. Laboratory studies suggest that the selection of appropriate types of antioxidants is crucial in terms of an optimal decrease in cancer incidence. For example, natural β-carotene reduces the frequency of radiation-induced transformation of normal cells in culture, whereas synthetic β-carotene does not. Beta-carotene induces certain biological effects that cannot be produced by vitamin A and vice versa. Beta-carotene not only acts as a precursor to vitamin A but also has some unique effects. Therefore, both β-carotene (in its natural rather than its synthetic form) and vitamin A should be included in any multiple antioxidant preparation used in a cancer prevention trial. Similarly, α-TS is the most effective form of vitamin E in minimizing the growth of cancer cells in culture or in the whole organism. Furthermore, various organs in rats selectively accumulate natural forms of vitamin E over the synthetic form. Thus d-α-tocopheryl succinate, rather than d-α-tocopherol or d-α-tocopheryl acetate, should be used in any cancer prevention protocol using micronutrients. Finally, vitamin C in the form of calcium ascorbate rather than ascorbic acid should be used, to lessen the risk of upset stomach that occurs in some people taking high doses of ascorbic acid.

6. Increased consumption of green tea has been associated with decreased risk of several cancers; therefore, the daily consumption of green tea is important.

7. Increased mental stress is associated with a higher risk of chronic diseases, including cancer. Adopting a lifestyle of reduced stress is an important component of cancer prevention.

It is clear from these conclusions that a definitive study is needed to assess the role of multiple micronutrients, together with modifications in diet and lifestyle. Furthermore, such a potential study must be performed among high-risk groups, and this would take at least five years. Results obtained from high-risk populations may not be fully applicable to normal, healthy people. Therefore, it is equally important to develop guidelines for cancer prevention in high-risk populations and guidelines for maintaining optimal health in healthy people. Any nutrients used for maintaining optimal health or for cancer prevention must satisfy the following criteria: (a) laboratory data on cancer prevention must be available for proposed micronutrients, and there must be a sound scientific rationale for using them, and (b) proposed micronutrients must be nontoxic at doses used.

How to Design Your Micronutrient Supplement, Diet, and Lifestyle Program to Reduce the Risk of Cancer

Several scientific agencies, such as the National Academy of Science, the American Cancer Society, and the American Institute for Cancer Research, have published dietary guidelines for reducing cancer risk. These contain very useful information but no recommendations for supplementary micronutrients. The Cancer Research Institute in New York also has prepared dietary guidelines that contain recommendations for micronutrients. Although there are no solid data from studies on human beings to suggest that supplemental β-carotene; vitamins A, C, and E; and selenium are essential for lowering the risk of cancer, there are sufficient animal and limited human studies that indicate that guidelines for supplementary micronutrients and minerals should be developed.

Proposed Guidelines for Micronutrient Supplements, Diet, and Lifestyle among the Normal Population to Maintain Optimal Health

Sustaining optimal health is essential for preventing such diseases as cancer. Free radicals are some of the primary toxins involved in raising the risk of cancer, heart disease, and neurological disease. If they damage normal dividing cells, the risk of cancer rises. If they damage nondividing cells, such as neurons, the risk of neurological diseases is enhanced. It follows that eliminating free radicals with antioxidants is important for supporting optimal health. It is also vital to obtain sufficient amounts of other nutrients, such as B vitamins and appropriate minerals.

Recommendations concerning the appropriate levels and types of micronutrients for the normal population depend upon age and gender. In some young women, anemia is an issue, owing to excessive loss of iron during menstruation. Anemia also develops during pregnancy in about 10 to 40 percent of women. A multiple micronutrient preparation containing vitamins A, C, and E; natural β-carotene; B vitamins; and appropriate minerals with no iron, copper, or manganese can be considered a baseline formulation for people of all age groups (men and women eighteen years and older). Since the biological half-life (time needed to reduce the nutrients in your body by half) of most micronutrients is about 6 to 12 hours, it is essential to take a supplement twice a day, half in the morning and half in the evening before meals. The reason for recommending taking supplements before meals is that many mutagens and carcinogens are formed during digestion. The presence of antioxidants in the gastrointestinal tract may curb the formation of these toxins. One appropriate multiple micronutrient preparation is available through the Rocky Mountain Medical Institute of Denver, Colorado, or Scientific Nutrition, Inc., in Oakland, California (1-800-990-7032).

Children should not be given supplemental micronutrients in the amounts recommended for an average adult. It is recommended that children take a multiple micronutrient supplement that is prepared using the same sound scientific rationale as that for adults. Rocky Mountain Medical Institute and Scientific Nutrition have these unique micronutrient preparations. The diet and lifestyle guidelines may be equally useful for children, except that the fat intake can be increased to about 30 percent of total calories. Small amounts of fiber can be consumed in the form of fruits, vegetables, and fiber-rich cereals.

Men and Women Aged Eighteen to Thirty-five Years

Supplements

Take an appropriately prepared multiple micronutrient supplement twice daily with a meal.

Diet Modifications

1. Eat three servings of fresh fruits and vegetables daily.

2. Consume about 26 g of fiber per day in the form of fruits, vegetables, and fiber-rich cereals.

3. Limit fat consumption to 20 percent of total calories (1 g of fat equals 9 calories). The current average fat consumption in the United States is 40 percent of calories from fat.

4. Avoid excessive protein, carbohydrates, and calories.

5. Restrict foods with high nitrate or nitrite content. Whenever eating such foods, take an antioxidant supplement before

the meal (or drink fresh orange juice before eating these foods).

6. Avoid eating large amounts of charcoal-broiled or smoked meat or fish.

7. Reduce the amount of pickled fruits and vegetables in the diet.

8. Curb consumption of caffeine-containing beverages (cold or hot).

Breakfast

- Whole wheat toast or fiber-rich cereals with low-fat or skim milk
- Fruits rich in β-carotene, such as apricots, mangoes, peaches, or cantaloupe
- Fruits rich in vitamin C, such as oranges, pineapples, strawberries, or raspberries

Lunch

- One piece (4 ounces) of skinless chicken or other low-fat meat or fish (not more than 4 ounces)
- Rolls, toast, or rice
- Fruits (same as those suggested for breakfast)
- Two vegetables (asparagus, spinach, broccoli, cabbage, corn, cauliflower, peas, beans, brussels sprouts, or potatoes)
- Salad containing spinach, parsley, cucumbers, and tomatoes, with a small amount of olive oil, low-fat salad dressing, or lemon juice

Dinner

The same suggestions as for lunch apply to dinner. In addition, one may eat any two fruits, one glass of low-fat or skim milk, and a low-calorie dessert.

Lifestyle Modifications

1. Avoid drinking excessive amounts of alcohol and caffeine-rich beverages.

2. DO NOT SMOKE. Avoid exposure to secondhand smoke. Do not chew tobacco.

3. Exercise 3 to 5 days a week for 30 minutes. If you do aerobic exercise for 30 minutes or more, take antioxidant supplements beforehand.

4. Adopt a lifestyle of limited stress.

5. Avoid overexposure to the sun. Do not use UV light for skin tanning or hyperbaric therapy for energy.

Men and Women Aged Thirty-six to Fifty Years

Supplements

Take an appropriately prepared multiple micronutrient supplement, as described for people aged eighteen to thirty-five. Take an additional 200 IU of vitamin E in the form of d-α-tocopheryl succinate and 1 g of vitamin C in the form of calcium ascorbate, divided into two doses.

To reduce the risk of osteoporosis, women should take an appropriate calcium-magnesium preparation with a small amount of vitamin D (1,500 mg calcium and 750 mg magnesium in the form of citrate, 100 IU of vitamin D), divided into two doses. These forms of calcium and magnesium are absorbed efficiently. Forms such as calcium oxide or magnesium oxide are not absorbed. Small amounts of vitamin D enhance the absorption of calcium from the intestinal tract. In addition, it is wise to eat a diet rich in foods that contain calcium, such as skim milk.

Diet and Lifestyle Guidelines

Dietary and lifestyle guidelines are the same as those described for people eighteen to thirty-five years of age.

Men and Women Aged Fifty-one to Sixty-five Years
Supplements

Take an appropriately prepared multiple micronutrient supplement, as described for people eighteen to thirty-five years old. Take an additional 200 IU of vitamin E in the form of *d*-α-tocopheryl succinate, an additional 2 g of vitamin C in the form of calcium ascorbate (divided into two doses), 30 mg of coenzyme Q10 twice a day, and 250 mg of NAC per day. The addition of coenzyme Q10 may be important in this age group, because it can improve mitochondrial function and thus increase energy levels. The likelihood of mitochondrial damage rises at this age. Glutathione levels in the body decrease with aging. *N*-acetylcysteine raises the levels of glutathione in the body, whereas glutathione itself does not. Women at this age should take a calcium-magnesium supplement, as described for women aged thirty-six to fifty. The loss of calcium increases with age, especially after menopause.

Diet and Lifestyle Guidelines

Dietary and lifestyle guidelines are the same as those described for people aged eighteen to thirty-five years.

Men and Women Older Than Sixty-five Years
Supplements

Take an appropriately prepared multiple micronutrient supplement, as described for people aged eighteen to thirty-five years. Take an additional 400 IU of vitamin E in the form of *d*-α-tocopheryl succinate, an additional 2 g of vitamin C in the form of calcium ascorbate (divided into two doses), 30 mg of coenzyme Q10 twice a day, 250 mg of NAC twice a day, and 15 mg of zinc per day. High doses (800 mg/day or more) of NAC increase the excretion of zinc in the urine. For this reason, a zinc supplement is recommended. The addition of coenzyme Q10 may be important for people in this age group, because it can improve mitochondrial function and increase energy levels. The likelihood of mitochondrial damage increases at this age. The SH compounds, such as glutathione, are important antioxidants that protect cells against free radical damage. Glutathione levels appear to decline slowly with advancing age, but glutathione cannot be taken as a supplement, because it is destroyed in the gut. Therefore, NAC, which is only partially destroyed in the gut and which raises the cellular levels of glutathione, is recommended for this group of people, as it was for those aged fifty-one to sixty-five. Women at this age should take a calcium-magnesium supplement, as described for women aged thirty-six to fifty.

Diet and Lifestyle Guidelines
Dietary and lifestyle guidelines are the same as those described for the group aged eighteen to thirty-five.

Proposed Guidelines for Micronutrient Supplements, Diet, and Lifestyle Among High-Risk Populations for Cancer Prevention

High-risk populations include heavy tobacco users, people with a family history of cancer, patients who are in remission from cancer, and patients with precancerous lesions (surgically removed or not removed). In terms of supplement recommendations, people at high risk can be divided into two groups: (a) heavy tobacco users and people with a familial history of cancer and (b) patients in remission from cancer and those with precancerous lesions.

Heavy Tobacco Users and People with a Family History of Cancer
Supplements
Take an appropriately prepared multiple micronutrient supplement, as described for people aged eighteen to thirty-five years.

Take an additional 400 IU of vitamin E in the form of *d*-α-tocopheryl succinate, an additional 2 g of vitamin C in the form of calcium ascorbate (divided into two doses), 15 mg of natural β-carotene per day, and 100 mcg of selenium per day. Women older than thirty-five should take a calcium-magnesium supplement, as described for women aged thirty-six to fifty.

Diet and Lifestyle Guidelines
Dietary and lifestyle guidelines are the same as those described for people aged eighteen to thirty-five, with the exception that the diet should derive not more than 15 percent of calories from fat.

Patients in Remission from Cancer and Patients with Precancerous Lesions

Supplements
Take an appropriately prepared multiple micronutrient supplement, as described for people aged eighteen to thirty-five. Take an additional 400 IU of vitamin E in the form of *d*-α-tocopheryl succinate, an additional 4 g of vitamin C in the form of calcium ascorbate (divided into two doses), 30 mg of natural β-carotene (divided into two doses), and 100 mcg of selenium. It is recommended that women take a calcium-magnesium supplement, as described for women aged thirty-six to fifty.

Diet and Lifestyle Guidelines
Dietary and lifestyle guidelines are the same as those as described for the group of people eighteen to thirty-five-years old. The fat content of the diet should be no more than 15 percent of calories. A lower fat level is recommended, because some patients in remission may have clinically undetectable cancers.

It should be emphasized that no clinical studies have been undertaken to assess the proposed guidelines for micronutrient supplements together with modifications in diet and lifestyle.

Therefore, it is advisable to consult a doctor before adopting the proposed guidelines. There has been no evidence to suggest that the doses of individual nutrients proposed in the guidelines are toxic to humans.

Additional Benefits of Following Cancer Prevention Guidelines

Adapting one's diet, taking supplementary micronutrients, and modifying one's lifestyle for cancer prevention is not limited to cancer protection. Such a program also may be very useful for supporting optimal health, because certain antioxidants can protect the body against injurious effects of agents that do not cause cancer. For example, accidental consumption of large amounts of mercury compounds has induced severe neurological diseases in human beings. Lower doses of mercury compounds may cause behavioral disturbances. Some laboratory experiments suggest that vitamin E reduces the risk of neurological diseases when supplemental antioxidants are given to animals during exposure to mercury compounds.

The generation of excess free radicals can lead to damage to dividing cells and increase the risk of cancer. When free radicals damage nondividing cells, such as nerve cells in the brain, they can raise the risk of neurological diseases. The presence of β-carotene; vitamins A, C, and E; and selenium in the body in sufficient amounts may protect these organs against the injurious effects of free radicals. Some scientists have proposed that an imbalance between the amounts of free radicals and certain antioxidants, such as β-carotene; vitamins A, C, and E; glutathione; and selenium, may be responsible for the normal aging process (i.e., more free radicals and fewer antioxidants may increase the rate of aging). If this is the case, the presence of sufficient amounts of these nutrients may lessen the damage and thereby reduce the rate of some degenerative changes associated with aging, especially in the brain. The proposed changes in diet, lifestyle, and supplementary micronutrients may also decrease the risk of heart disease and eye diseases, such as cataracts, since free radicals also play a major role in the development of these diseases. Several human studies have shown that supplementation with vitamin E lowers the risk of heart disease. Another study found that supplementation with antioxidants also lessens the risk of cataract.

Guidelines for Selecting Micronutrients

Cautions

1. In recent years, many nutrition books have been published, and some contain erroneous information regarding doses and dose schedules for supplementary nutrients. It is important to select the book by which to prepare your diet guidelines carefully. Make sure that the credentials of the authors include research, patient care, and teaching expertise in the area of vitamins and nutrition.

2. Base your estimate of vitamins and nutrients for daily consumption on your needs, and check with a physician who is knowledgeable in this area to see whether your estimates are reasonable.

3. Do not buy any vitamins or nutrients that are not fully described on the label.

4. Do not take excessive amounts of nutrients. Some nutrition books have suggested that one should increase the doses

until side effects or illness become evident and then decrease the doses until a comfortable level is reached. This method is very dangerous, because some nutrients in large amounts can cause irreversible damage.

5. If you have further questions, consult experts who are actively involved in research, teaching, or patient care (see the appendix).

These considerations will make your efforts to improve your health and reduce the risk of cancer more effective and less expensive. Reliable scientific information regarding micronutrients is available through the Rocky Mountain Medical Institute or Scientific Nutrition.

Specifics

Based on your age, sex, and health status, determine your need for supplemental nutrition with respect to type, chemical form, and dose of each micronutrient before going to any health food store. Consult your doctor. Be cautious about advice suggested in commercial advertisements (through TV, radio, newspapers, magazines, or health food store personnel).

Selecting a multiple micronutrient formula is difficult, because the individual micronutrients (with respect to dose, chemical form, and number) markedly vary, not only from one company to another but also within the same company. Unfortunately, no justification is ever given, except that they are good for you. A few examples will demonstrate the point that adequate attention is not paid to the rationale for adding a particular ingredient. For example, inositol, a very important chemical for cellular function, is added to some multiple vitamin preparations in the amount of 30 to 50 mg. If you know that 1,000 mg of inositol is consumed every day through the diet, the addition of such a small amount of inositol can be considered a commercial gimmick with no health benefits. Similar statements can be made with respect to adding choline and methionine to any multiple vitamin preparation.

Make sure the preparation has no iron, copper, or manganese and no heavy metals, such as boron, vanadium, and molybdenum, and that it contains both vitamin A and β-carotene (natural) at appropriate doses, two forms of vitamin E (d-α-tocopherol and d-α-TS), vitamin C as calcium ascorbate, B vitamins (not more than two to three times the RDA), and appropriate doses of such minerals as selenium, zinc, and chromium. The antioxidants coenzyme Q10, NAC, and NADH may be beneficial for patients with heart disease and neurological diseases, but they may be detrimental to patients undergoing radiation therapy or chemotherapy. N-acetylcysteine, for example, has been shown to protect both cancer cells and normal cells against the damaging effects of radiation therapy and chemotherapy. A multiple micronutrient preparation should contain those antioxidants that are useful under all conditions. They include vitamin A, β-carotene, vitamins C and E, and selenium.

Concluding Remarks

Laboratory and human studies suggest that multiple micronutrients, as well as modifications in diet and lifestyle, may lower the risk of cancer. These three factors are equally important in cancer prevention. Adopting one alone may not be optimally effective. Studies also show that the use of a single micronutrient in any cancer prevention trial has no scientific merit. Such a trial may produce no effect or a small benefit, or it may have a harmful effect. Human epidemiological studies should not be interpreted as conclusive until laboratory data confirm the conclusions. Most of the confusion is created when the results of epidemiological investigations are considered to be conclusive rather than as raising important questions that must be answered by intervention trials in human and laboratory experiments.

Based on laboratory and human studies, we have proposed guidelines for micronutrient supplements as well as for diet and lifestyle modifications for optimal health and for cancer prevention. This guideline will be modified whenever new scientific data become available. We have emphasized the use of appropriate micronutrients, including antioxidants, B vitamins, and minerals, with respect to dose, type, and chemical form. It is hoped that the proposed guidelines will help consumers select the right kinds of supplements and ask questions if they have any doubts about them.

6 Antioxidants in Combination with Standard Therapy in the Treatment of Cancer

Before discussing the role of multiple micronutrients in combination with standard therapy in the treatment of cancer, we will outline the nature of cancer cells and the present status, usefulness, and limitations of standard and experimental cancer therapy.

Are All Cells of a Particular Cancer Similar?

If all cells of a specific type of cancer were similar, treating cancer would be easier, because one therapeutic agent would kill all the cells. Unfortunately, cancer cells are very complex in the sense that there are many different kinds of cells with respect to their sensitivity to drugs, even within the same cancer. Therefore, several drugs that have different modes of action typically are used in treating cancer. Such drugs are called *chemotherapeutic agents.* Chemotherapeutic agents in combination kill more cancer cells than would be killed by a single agent.

It has been observed repeatedly that cancer cells may become unresponsive to all therapeutic agents after a period of good initial response. This finding stems from the fact that almost all the agents used to treat cancer can cause cancer themselves. During treatment, these agents produce many biochemical changes among those cancer cells that are not killed and make them "super cancer cells." These cancer cells become very resistant to all chemotherapeutic agents and radiation.

To summarize, tumor cells may be different from one another; some differences are inherent (i.e., they are present before treatment), whereas other differences are acquired (i.e., they are generated by treatment agents). We can clearly see that the complexity of tumor cells increases during the treatment phase and that no single agent may ever be sufficient to cure cancers.

Benefits and Limitations of Various Treatments

Current standard cancer therapies include surgery, chemotherapy, radiation therapy, and experimental therapies, including heat therapy, immunotherapy, and gene therapy. Frequently, surgery is used in combination with chemotherapy and radiation or in combination with chemotherapy, radiation, and heat. The usefulness and limitations of each of these therapeutic agents are discussed here.

Surgery
Surgery is one of the most common procedures in the treatment of solid cancers. Many cancer sites are not accessible, however; even when they are, some cancer cells are often left in the body. Nevertheless, surgery is considered one of the best available approaches to cancer therapy, because it does not significantly increase the risk of new cancers or noncancerous diseases.

Chemotherapy

Many toxic chemicals are used extensively in treating cancer, frequently in combination with surgery and radiation. Almost all of them kill both cancer cells and normal cells, cause severe illness, destroy the body's immune defense system, and raise the risk of new cancer among patients who survive more than five years. In addition, the efficacy of chemotherapy has reached a plateau for the treatment of many human solid cancers. It is especially ineffective for the treatment of melanoma (a type of skin tumor), brain tumors, and lung cancer. Therefore, additional approaches must be developed to improve the efficacy of chemotherapy.

Reports show that the incidence of leukemia (blood cancer) and solid tumors among the survivors of chemotherapy and radiation therapy is about 10 percent, but the observation periods upon which this figure is based are usually no more than ten years after completion of treatment. According to present knowledge, the risk of leukemia may not increase further ten years after treatment, but the risk of new solid cancers and noncancerous diseases persists up to thirty years or more after treatment. In spite of these limitations, chemotherapy must be used until better treatment methods are established.

Radiation Therapy

Radiation, in the form of X- and gamma-irradiation, is a typical treatment for many types of human cancer. Occasionally, neutron radiation is used. The advantage of neutron radiation is that it can kill those tumor cells that are normally resistant to X-irradiation. The disadvantage of neutron radiation is that it is more damaging to normal cells than X-radiation. Radiation therapy is frequently used in combination with surgery or chemotherapy or both. Some tumors, such as childhood leukemia, Hodgkin lymphoma, testicular embryonal carcinoma, and neuroblastoma, respond to radiation therapy very well, whereas other tumors, such as melanoma, respond very poorly.

Like chemotherapy, radiation has toxic effects. It kills both normal and cancer cells, causes severe illness, destroys the body's immune defense system, and increases the risk of new cancer among those who survive. Generally, the time interval between radiation exposure and detection of new tumors is about ten years for leukemia and up to thirty years or more for solid tumors. The risk of noncancerous diseases, such as aplastic anemia, or delayed necrosis in organs containing non-dividing cells (such as the brain and liver) also persists after completion of treatment (usually more than fifteen years). In spite of these limitations, radiation must be used until better treatment methods are established. Agents that can protect normal cells selectively without protecting cancer cells, or agents that enhance the effect of irradiation on cancer cells but not on normal cells, would improve the efficacy of radiation treatment.

Hyperthermia (Heat Therapy)

Tumor cells are more sensitive to heat than normal cells with respect to growth inhibition. Heat therapy was discovered accidentally in 1893, when cancer patients of Dr. Coley of Columbia University experienced high temperatures owing to infection. Since antibiotics had not been discovered yet, these high temperatures persisted for a few days. Dr. Coley observed that some of the tumors of patients with fevers shrank markedly. This remarkable discovery remained in relative obscurity until the 1960s, when radiation biologists re-investigated heat therapy. At present, temperatures of 42–43°C (107.6–109.4°F) are commonly used in heat therapy, primarily for the purpose of controlling local tumors.

Heat therapy is given when all standard therapy has failed. Raising the whole-body temperature from 37°C (98.6°F) to 42°C or 43°C even for a short time can cause severe adverse effects.

However, heat often is used in combination with radiation therapy. This approach has provided occasional relief for some patients when other treatment methods have proved ineffective, but, in general, results of heat therapy have been disappointing. Some recent laboratory experiments suggest that the use of high temperatures (42–43°C) in combination with radiation actually may increase the risk of radiation-induced cancer. Because of these limitations, the use of such high temperatures cannot be considered in designing long-term heat treatment strategies for human cancer. Whole-body heat therapy at a lower temperature (40°C, or 104°F), in combination with nontoxic chemicals that increase the effect of heat, may be of great value in treating human cancer, because the whole-body temperature can be raised from 37°C to 40°C without toxic effects. Heat therapy should be given at the beginning rather than at the end of standard therapy.

Immunotherapy

Monoclonal antibodies to specific cellular proteins are produced by biotechnology companies. It is assumed that such monoclonal antibodies will help kill cancer cells that bind to these antibodies. Unfortunately, these antibodies are not specific for cancer cells; they also can bind with many normal cells. Thus, the usefulness of such antibodies in treating cancer is limited. Antibodies obtained from the heat-shock protein of tumor cells selectively kill tumor cells without affecting normal cells. Such antibodies have shown some beneficial effects on certain human tumors. A large clinical study on this issue is lacking, however. Certain types of bacteria, and even a patient's own tumor cells, are inactivated for use in immunotherapy. Varying degrees of tumor regression have been observed with this treatment.

In addition, attempts have been made to make a patient's own natural killer cells more efficient through genetic engineering. Such immunotherapy also has caused varying degrees of tumor regression. Appropriate immunotherapy remains one of the potentially most useful strategies in cancer therapy. Extensive laboratory studies are in progress to evaluate the efficacy of various immunotherapies.

Gene Therapy

This therapy involves the delivery of toxic genes to tumor cells or the drug targeting of mutated genes that are present only in cancer cells. Theoretically, gene therapy selectively kills cancer cells. The major limitation has been gene delivery to the target tumor tissue. The few clinical trials have not shown encouraging results; for this reason, the role of gene therapy in the management of human tumors remains elusive. Extensive laboratory and clinical studies are being conducted to clarify this issue.

Anti-Angiogenesis Drug Therapy

This therapy entails use of a drug that inhibits angiogenesis (the formation of blood vessels). As tumors grow, new vascular systems are formed in order to derive nutrition for survival. It once was thought that an anti-angiogenesis drug would inhibit the formation of blood vessels and thus starve the tumor to death. Indeed, anti-angiogenesis drugs have cured tumors in mice. This was an excellent idea; unfortunately, clinical trials with anti-angiogenesis drugs have not been encouraging, owing to the drugs' toxicities. Efforts must be made to develop anti-angiogenesis drugs that are nontoxic. Such drugs would cause selective tumor regression. A recent study has shown that α-TS may act as an anti-angiogenesis agent in animal tumor models.

Delayed Consequences of Cancer Therapies

Treatment methods available at present have produced growing numbers of long-term survivors of early-stage diseases, such as Hodgkin disease, childhood leukemia, Wilms tumor (affecting the kidney), cervical cancer, prostate cancer, neuroblastoma, retinoblastoma (an eye tumor), and melanoma (skin cancer). There is a risk that new cancers and noncancerous diseases will develop in these "cured" patients. In the case of most other cancers, current treatment agents have been less effective.

Based on five-year survival rates, significant progress has been made in the treatment of some cancers. But if one considers recent indications of a growing risk of new cancers and noncancer diseases, one becomes concerned about the consequences and adequacy of available methods of treatment. Noncancerous diseases that may afflict survivors include the following:

- Aplastic anemia, if the bone marrow was targeted by therapy
- Paralysis, if the spinal cord was involved in therapy
- Cataracts, if one or both eyes were affected by therapy
- Reproductive failures, if the reproductive organs were involved in therapy
- Necrosis in nondividing organs, such as the brain and muscle cells, if they were affected by therapy
- Retardation of growth if the patient was a child

Because of these potential risks, newer approaches to cancer treatments that utilize nontoxic agents must be developed. It should be emphasized, however, that present methods of treatment must continue despite potential risks until better therapies are available.

Better Methods of Cancer Treatment

The best way to treat cancer would be to convert all cancer cells into cells that are more like normal cells that are noncancerous or to kill all cancer cells without killing normal cells or both. To achieve the first goal, we need to understand the basic steps in maintaining the regular features of normal cells and the fundamental events that lead to malignant transformation of normal cells. To achieve the second goal, we must identify substances that kill cancer cells without killing normal cells. If one considers the evolution of cancer cells in the body, it is possible, in theory, to discover nontoxic agents that can change cancer cells to more normal cells and that can kill only tumor cells. For example, the conversion from normal cells to cancer cells probably occurs more frequently than we realize; however, these newly formed cancer cells do not always develop into detectable cancer, possibly because the body has an elaborate defense system, which includes the immune system and antioxidant systems. When cancer cells escape these defense systems, tumor cells establish themselves in the host and grow.

Micronutrient Therapy

Micronutrients include certain antioxidants, B vitamins, and appropriate minerals. Antioxidants such as vitamins A, C, and E and carotenoids play a part in differentiation and growth inhibition of cancer cells, as we have seen. Other micronutrients, such as B vitamins and minerals, are depleted during radiation and chemotherapy. Therefore, it is essential to combine all of these micronutrients, rather than antioxidants alone, with standard therapy. Numerous laboratory experiments in cell cultures and in animals, in addition to some human studies, indicate that certain micronutrients, such as β-carotene and vitamins A, C, and E, can change some cancer cells back to more normal cells, which are non–tumor forming (the process called *differentiation*). They also kill cancer cells without killing normal cells. Antioxidants in combination are more effective than individual antioxidants in limiting the growth of tumor cells. The following sections describe the importance of antioxidants alone or in combination with prevalent tumor therapeutic agents.

Laboratory experiments suggest that micronutrients may improve cancer treatment markedly in the following ways:

1. Reduce tumor growth without affecting normal cells

2. Convert some cancer cells into cells that are like normal

3. Enhance the cell-killing effects of currently used chemotherapeutic agents and radiation and heat therapies

4. Lessen some of the toxic side effects of irradiation and chemotherapeutic agents on normal cells

5. Stimulate the body's immune defense system

The extent and type of these effects depend upon the type, form, dosage, and method of administration of micronutrients as well as the type and stage of the tumor. We will now look at the importance of high-dose individual micronutrients in treating cancer.

Beta-carotene and Vitamin A

Both β-carotene and vitamin A (13-*cis*-retinoic acid, other analogs of retinoic acid) inhibit the growth of some cancer cells in culture. They also convert some cancer cells to cells that are like normal. Beta-carotene at a dose of 180 mg per week effected complete remission in 15 percent of patients with oral leukoplakia, a potentially premalignant lesion. The combination of β-carotene and vitamin A (100,000 IU per week) caused complete remission in 27 percent of those patients. compared with a placebo group, in which complete remission was observed in only 3 percent. A higher dose of vitamin A alone (13-*cis*-retinoic acid at 200,000 IU per week) led to complete remission in 27 percent of patients with oral leukoplakia.

The recurrence of melanoma after surgical removal of the primary tumor is high (30 to 75 percent), depending upon the stage of the cancer. Reports show that the combination of BCG vaccine with vitamin A (100,000 IU per day), taken for eighteen months, slightly increases the disease-free period in stages I and II melanoma compared with BCG vaccine alone. The side effects of this treatment included dry skin and mild depression. The administration of BCG alone has produced varying degrees of tumor regression. One of the actions of BCG is stimulation of the immune system.

A pronounced beneficial effect of 13-*cis*-retinoic acid on cutaneous T-cell lymphoma (mycosis fungoides) has been observed. In one study, eight of twelve patients responded well, and four of the twelve showed signs of nearly complete cure. Beneficial effects of vitamin A were also noted in patients with epithelial tumors. Some epithelial tumor cells are resistant to vitamin A; the reasons for their resistance are unknown. Vitamin A was ineffective in treating nonepithelial cancer.

Further studies are needed to evaluate the role of high-dose β-carotene and vitamin A in the treatment of human cancers. It is certain that β-carotene and vitamin A by themselves are not sufficient in the treatment of advanced cancer. In addition, the toxicity of vitamin A in doses of 100,000–200,000 IU may be a limiting factor. However, laboratory data show that if vitamin A and β-carotene are used together in multiple micronutrient preparations, the effective dose requirements may be lower. Individually, retinoids or β-carotene at low doses can stimulate the growth of certain cancer cells. For this and other reasons, the use of a single micronutrient in cancer treatment has no scientific merit.

Vitamin C

Although vitamin C has been shown to reduce the growth of animal tumors, its role in treating human cancer has become controversial. The researchers Cameron and Pauling have reported that the administration of high doses of sodium ascorbate (5 to

10 g per day) lengthens the survival time of patients with advanced cancer. These patients either were treated minimally with conventional therapies or were not treated at all. Other scientists have reported that high doses of vitamin C were ineffective in improving the survival of patients with terminal cancer. These patients were treated extensively with radiation therapy and chemotherapy before vitamin C treatment was started. The reasons for the difference in results of these studies are not known, but the patient groups in the two studies were different.

Vitamin C at low doses can stimulate the growth of some cancer cells, such as certain cancers of the salivary gland. Therefore, vitamin C alone may not be useful for the long-term management of human cancer. It is interesting to note that in alternative medicine practices, vitamin C in doses as high as 80 g are given intravenously to patients with advanced disease who have failed all treatments. Claims have been made of a beneficial effect of this treatment on tumor regression, without toxicity. We do not recommend this treatment until a control trial on the value of injected high-dose vitamin C shows a beneficial effect on tumor regression in advanced stages of cancer.

One study has reported that local infusion of sodium ascorbate with copper and glycyl-glycyl-histidine, a peptide (protein), caused complete regression of osteosarcoma (bone cancer) in one patient. This interesting observation calls for further research. We should point out, however, that high-dose vitamin C alone may never be sufficient treatment of human cancer.

Vitamin E

Laboratory experiments have shown that α-TS-tocopheryl succinate causes some cancer cells to revert to normal-appearing cells and inhibits the growth of several other cancer cells. At similar doses, other forms of vitamin E, such as α-tocopherol, α-tocopheryl acetate, and α-tocopheryl nicotinate, were ineffective. However, cancer cells that are resistant to α-TS do exist, and the reasons for their resistance are unknown. The extent and type of effect of vitamin E on cancer cells depend upon the form of cancer and the form of vitamin E. Alpha-tocopheryl succinate has inhibited the growth of transplanted tumors or chemical-induced tumors in animals, and it exhibited anti-angiogenesis activity in the animal tumor models. This is an important finding, because, unlike other anti-angiogenesis drugs, α-TS is nontoxic in humans.

In one clinical trial, high doses of α-tocopherol were used to treat human neuroblastoma that had become unresponsive to all standard therapeutic agents. Studies showed that more than 50 percent of these patients showed partial regression of the cancer. We should point out that the α-tocopherol that was used in this study may not be the most potent form of vitamin E. In view of the fact that patients who received vitamin E therapy were terminally ill and became unresponsive to all available therapy, these preliminary results should be considered encouraging. Vitamin E also causes regression of oral leukoplakia in humans.

High doses of α-TS must be added to any micronutrient therapy. In clinical or experimental studies, researchers must consider. the type of vitamin E (α-TS is the most active type), the form of vitamin E (cells preferentially take up the natural form of vitamin E, or the *d* form), and the dose and dose schedule (800 IU divided into two doses).

Combined Antioxidants

Because of the presence of different kinds of cells in a cancer and because β-carotene and vitamins A, C, and E have different modes of action, the combination of these four micronutrients may be more effective in the treatment of cancer than the individual micronutrients alone. Indeed, laboratory data suggest that multiple micronutrients (vitamins A, C, and E and β-carotene) are more effective than single micronutrients in limiting the growth of tumor cells in cell culture. In a recent human study, the combination of vitamins A, C, and E lessened the rate of cell proliferation in colon mucosa (the lining of the colon). No human studies have been undertaken to assess the efficacy of several micronutrients in slowing tumor growth. Because of the potential for enhancement of tumor growth at low doses of individual antioxidants, we do not recommend the use of a single nutrient in cancer treatment.

Vitamin B$_6$

Some animal studies have reported that supplemental vitamin B$_6$, one of the vitamins of the B complex, enhances the growth of human breast cancer transplanted into athymic mice (mice with no thymus gland) and that the restriction of vitamin B$_6$ retards it. The relevance of this observation to human cancer is not known at this time. Nevertheless, supplementation with high doses of vitamin B$_6$ (50 mg/day or more) should be avoided during treatment of breast cancer; however, low doses of B$_6$ (less than 10 mg/day) are needed, because radiation therapy and chemotherapy decrease the levels of micronutrients, including B vitamins.

Vitamin D

Recent laboratory experiments show that 1-α-hydroxyvitamin D$_3$ (a form of vitamin D) reduces the growth in cell culture of certain cancers, for example, melanoma, hepatocellular carcinoma (a liver cancer), and myeloid leukemia (a kind of blood cancer). It also converts some cancer cells, such as human leukemia cells, to cells that are more like normal in culture. Because of the toxicity of vitamin D, however, we do not recommend high doses of this vitamin during cancer treatment.

The mechanisms of action by which β-carotene and vitamins A, C, D, and E curb growth or induce differentiation (conversion of cancer cells to cells that are more like normal) in cancer cells are not known. Normal cells may have membrane systems that prevent excessive uptake of these micronutrients in spite of their high levels in the blood. This important membrane system in cancer cells becomes defective, however, which then allows the entry of large amounts of micronutrients. In larger amounts, these micronutrients may trigger a series of genetic changes that can cause growth inhibition and cell differentiation in tumor cells. These genetic changes are described in chapter 5. Such changes do not occur in micronutrient-treated normal cells, and thus micronutrients do not cause growth inhibition in normal cells. Based on experimental data, it is clear that even multiple micronutrients by themselves are not adequate to treat human cancer effectively.

Enhancement of the Effects of Tumor Therapeutic Agents by Beta-carotene and Vitamins A, C, and E

Results of laboratory experiments indicate that high-dose β-carotene and vitamins A, C, and E can intensify the growth-inhibitory effects of therapeutic agents (chemotherapy, radiation, and heat) on cancer cells. The extent of enhancement depends upon the types of tumor cells, the types of micronutrients, and the types of cancer-therapeutic agents. Therapeutic agents can be grouped into these categories: radiation, surgery, chemotherapeutic agents, naturally occurring anticancer agents, and heat. The enhancement of the effects of such treatments by micronutrients is discussed in the following sections.

Enhancement of the Beneficial Effects of X-irradiation and Chemotherapeutic Agents on Tumor Cells with High-dose Vitamin A and Beta-carotene

Animal studies suggest that vitamin A and β-carotene inhibit the growth of breast cancer in animals. Vitamin A together with radiation or β-carotene with radiation produced a cure rate of more than 90 percent. Cancers were completely cured in mice given both vitamin A and radiation. The combination of cyclophosphamide, a commonly used chemotherapeutic agent, with vitamin A or β-carotene effected a similar level of cure in animals with transplanted breast cancer. This study suggests that combining β-carotene and vitamin A with certain therapeutic agents can improve the results of cancer treatment.

Retinoids enhance the cytotoxicity of cisplatin on human ovarian cancer cells transplanted into athymic mice. Retinoid plus interferon alpha-2a augmented radiation-induced damage of head and neck squamous cell carcinoma cells in culture. This antioxidant also enhances the effect of interferon alpha-2a on squamous cell carcinoma cells of the cervix. Retinoic acid in combination with tamoxifen inhibits the growth of human melanoma cells in culture more than individual agents alone. Retinoic acid also has heightened the effects of irradiation on cancer cells in culture. Because of the toxicity of high-dose retinoids in humans, we do not recommend the use of this micronutrient alone in combination with standard therapy.

Enhancement of the Benefits of X-irradiation and Chemotherapeutic Agents on Tumor Cells with High-dose Vitamin C

Studies have shown that high-dose vitamin C increases the effects of irradiation and several chemotherapeutic agents on neuroblastoma cells. Vitamin C in combination with irradiation lengthens the survival of mice with tumor cells growing in the fluid of the abdominal cavity more than irradiation alone. Moreover, vitamin C protects hamster ovary cells against radiation damage. High-dose vitamin C by itself was ineffective against radiation damage of glioma cells (a form of brain tumor) in culture. One study has shown that vitamin C (sodium ascorbate) in combination with CCNU (a commonly used chemotherapeutic agent) enhances the survival of mice with leukemia twofold, compared with results obtained when CCNU is used alone. High-dose vitamin C heightens the effect of several other chemotherapeutic agents, such as 5-fluorouracil, adriamycin, bleomycin, and vincristine, on neuroblastoma cells in culture. Some investigators have indicated that high doses of vitamin C should not be given in conjunction with radiation therapy or chemotherapy. This suggestion is based on studies in which radioactive vitamin C accumulated more in tumor cells growing in animals than in the brain tissue of the same animals. Such a recommendation has no scientific merit in the absence of experimental results using vitamin C with radiation or with chemotherapeutic agents.

Enhancement of the Beneficial Effects of X-irradiation and Chemotherapeutic Agents on Tumor Cells with Vitamin E

Laboratory experiments have shown that high doses of vitamin E (α-TS and the aqueous form of α-tocopheryl acetate) increase the effects of irradiation on neuroblastoma cells, glioma cells (brain tumor), human cervical cancer cells, and human ovarian cancer cells, whereas low doses of vitamin E are ineffective. Vitamin E succinate, however, does not enhance the effect of irradiation on normal human cells in culture. Vitamin E succinate also amplifies the effect of many chemotherapeutic agents on several tumor cells in culture and in animals. One study has shown that the aqueous form of vitamin E was more effective in limiting the growth of human colon cancer cells transplanted into athymic mice than 5-fluorouracil (5-FU) alone. The combination of vitamin E and 5-FU was much more potent than the individual agents in reducing the growth of tumor. These studies emphasize that the appropriate form of vitamin E must be used in any clinical trial for the treatment of cancer. As mentioned previously, we also advise using multiple rather than single micronutrients in combination with standard cancer therapy in the treatment of human cancer.

Enhancement of the Beneficial Effects of
Naturally Occurring Anticancer Agents with Vitamin E

The use of toxic drugs in treating human tumors continues to be emphasized, but it cannot be accepted as the ideal therapy. An alternative approach must be developed. Several studies indicate that it may be possible to treat human cancer with high doses of nontoxic, naturally occurring substances. These agents at higher concentrations convert some cancer cells to normal cells and/or reduce the growth of tumors without affecting normal cells.

In addition to antioxidants, two naturally occurring substances, cAMP and butyric acid (a very small fatty acid), have been found to induce growth inhibition and differentiation in several rodent and human cancer cells in culture and in humans. The chemical substance cAMP is found in all cells of the body. Several laboratory experiments have suggested that a defect in the cAMP system may be associated with the formation of some types of cancer cells. If this is the case, then the correction of this defect should convert cancer cells back to normal cells.

Indeed, when cAMP levels are elevated with the aid of another chemical, some tumor cells, such as neuroblastoma, melanoma, small-cell carcinoma (a lung cancer), glioma, and pheochromocytoma (an adrenal cancer), become more like normal cells. As expected, not all cancer cells are converted to normal cells by elevating cAMP levels. Additional studies must be performed to find out how the remaining cancer cells can be changed to normal cells. The finding that cancer cells can be selectively transformed in this way with cAMP-stimulating agents is very exciting, but the usefulness of this concept in treating human cancer has been tested in only one type of cancer (neuroblastoma). The addition of cAMP-stimulating agents to the treatment protocols for advanced neuroblastoma has shown encouraging results. Because of the toxicity of cAMP-stimulating agents, this approach is not promising.

We have shown that vitamin E succinate enhances the effect of cAMP on differentiation of neuroblastoma cells and melanoma cells in culture. This observation is very important, because it illustrates for the first time that vitamin E not only acts directly on some cancer cells but also intensifies the effects of other naturally occurring substances, such as cAMP.

Butyric acid, a small fatty acid, also occurs naturally in the human body. A high-fiber diet heightens the production of butyric acid in the lower colon as the result of fermentation of fiber by bacteria that are present in the colon. In laboratory experiments, butyric acid is used in the form sodium butyrate (nonacidic form). Numerous laboratory experiments have shown that sodium butyrate at high doses also transforms some cancer cells (erythroid leukemia, a cancer of blood cells) to cells that are more like normal. In addition, it kills other cancer cells without killing normal cells (for example, neuroblastoma, sarcoma, glioma, and melanoma cells). As expected, not all cancer cells are killed by sodium butyrate. We still must discover how the remaining cancer cells can be killed or converted to normal cells.

Limited human studies suggest that sodium butyrate at high doses (up to 10 g per day), administered intravenously, is nontoxic and has beneficial effects in some patients with advanced neuroblastomas and erythroid leukemia. The biological turnover of sodium butyrate in the body is rapid. It would be necessary, therefore, to develop analogs of butyric acid, which can maintain anticancer activity with increased stability. Because it selectively affects cancer cells, it is a very promising anticancer agent. Sodium butyrate also enhances the effect of X-irradiation and chemotherapeutic agents on tumor cells in culture. The combination of sodium butyrate and vitamin E succinate is more effective than the individual agents in limiting the growth of tumor cells in culture.

Enhancement of the Beneficial Effects of Heat Therapy on Cancer Cells with Vitamin E

During the past ten years, extensive experiments and clinical studies have been conducted on the effects of heat alone or in combination with X rays and certain chemotherapeutic agents, primarily for the treatment of local tumors. The results of clinical trials have been disappointing, however, because the temperatures used to kill cancer cells are 42–43°C and the human body cannot tolerate these temperatures without serious side effects. Even in the treatment of local lesions, heat has been of very limited value. In addition, such high temperatures increase the potential of X rays to cause cancer. The use of heat in the treatment of tumors will continue to be restricted to local lesions until the cell-killing effects of heat can be achieved at temperatures near 40°C, which are not toxic to the whole body.

At present, heat treatment is given at the end of standard therapy, when tumor cells become more resistant to X-irradiation and chemotherapeutic agents owing to the accumulation of a number of mutations. Killing resistant cells requires the use of high temperatures (42–43°C). Thus, the prevailing strategy of heat treatment has no biological rationale and will not have a significant impact on the management of human cancer. Alpha-tocopheryl succinate in combination with heat at 40°C was more effective than single agents in reducing the growth of neuroblastoma cells in culture. We believe that heat therapy can be very useful when it is given to the whole body at 40–41°C along with multiple micronutrients before the administration of X-irradiation or chemotherapeutic agents.

Micronutrients and Reduction of the Toxic Effects of Radiation Therapy and Chemotherapy on Normal Cells

Beta-carotene at high doses limited the severity of radiation-induced mucositis (soreness of the mouth) in humans during treatment of head and neck cancer. Vitamin E also curbed doxorubicin-induced damage to the liver, heart, kidneys, and intestines in normal animals. Alpha-tocopheryl succinate protects bone marrow against toxicity caused by azidothymidine in normal animals. Several animal studies have shown that vitamin E may limit the cardiac toxicity and skin ulcers produced by adriamycin. Vitamin E has been found to protect against bleomycin-induced lung fibrosis. Some studies showed that vitamin E defends the immune system against the destructive effect of several chemotherapeutic agents, such as adriamycin, mitomycin C, and 5-FU. These studies in normal animals show that vitamins can protect normal cells against damage caused by certain chemotherapeutic agents.

Vitamin E succinate failed to safeguard normal human fibroblasts (skin cells) against reductions in cell cycle movement (i.e., the growth rate) brought about by radiation, but it protected normal cells against radiation-induced chromosomal damage. It also has been reported that vitamin C (sodium ascorbate) significantly diminished adriamycin-induced heart damage in mice and guinea pigs. Calcitriol, a form of vitamin D, protects animals from alopecia (baldness) caused by chemotherapy. Human trials should be undertaken to test the efficacy of these micronutrients in lessening the adverse effects of radiation therapy and chemotherapy.

Micronutrients That Decrease the Effects of Radiation Therapy and Chemotherapy on Cancer Cells

When some antioxidants, such as SH compounds, are given before X-irradiation or treatment with chemotherapeutic agents, they produce effects on tumor cells that are opposite to those generated by such antioxidants as vitamins A, C, and E and carotenoids. Examples of SH compounds include glutathione and cysteine. Alpha-lipoic acid and NAC raise the intracellular levels of glutathione and protect both normal cells and cancer cells against radiation damage. As a matter of fact, differences in radiosensitivity of both normal and cancer cells as a function of cell cycle phase stem from differences in the levels of SH compounds.

All dividing normal cells and cancer cells pass through the various phases of the cell cycle: the pre-DNA synthetic phase, the DNA synthetic phase, the post-DNA synthetic phase, and the mitotic phase. It is well established that mitotic cells, which are the most sensitive to damage caused by irradiation, have the lowest levels of SH compounds. DNA synthetic phase cells, which are the most resistant to radiation-induced damage, have the highest levels of SH compounds. In addition, when the levels of SH compounds in mitotic cells were elevated experimentally, the cells became very resistant to radiation. SH compounds also may safeguard normal and cancer cells against the destructive effects of most chemotherapeutic agents. Therefore, the agents that increase the levels of SH compounds in both normal and cancer cells should never be used in combination with radiation therapy or chemotherapy.

In contrast to SH compounds, antioxidants such as vitamins A, C, and E and carotenoids strengthen the effects of standard therapeutic agents on cancer cells, but they actually may defend normal cells against some of these adverse effects. For this reason, data obtained on the effects of one antioxidant on cancer cells or normal cells should not be extrapolated to other antioxidants without experimental studies. Occasionally, vitamin C partially or completely blocks the damaging effects of DTIC and methotrexate (cancer therapeutic agents) on mouse neuroblastoma cells in culture. When the effects on human melanoma cells of vitamin C in combination with DTIC were studied, however, the growth inhibition was more pronounced than that of the individual agents. It also should be pointed out that when multiple micronutrients, such as vitamins A, C, and E and carotenoids, are used together with standard therapeutic agents, no protection of human cancer cells has ever been observed, provided that antioxidants are present before and during treatment and throughout the observation period. Removal of antioxidants immediately after exposure to therapeutic agents may cause adverse effects.

Enhanced Effectiveness of Multiple Antioxidants Compared with Single Antioxidants in Reducing the Growth of Cancer Cells

Individual antioxidants provoke varying degrees of growth inhibition in cancer cells developing in culture dishes or in vivo. Tumor regression in humans can be achieved at very high doses, which frequently cause toxicity, especially with retinoid derivatives. At lower doses they may be ineffective or may even stimulate the growth of cancer cells. Therefore, the use of single antioxidants in cancer treatment has no biological or clinical merit. Recent studies suggest that combination antioxidants are more effective in limiting the growth of human cancer and precancerous cells than single antioxidants. For example, a mixture of four antioxidants (13-*cis*-retinoic acid, *d*-α-tocopheryl succinate, vitamin C as sodium ascorbate, and a carotenoid) markedly slowed the growth of human melanoma cells in culture at doses at which each antioxidant alone had no effect on growth. This study suggests that lower doses of individual antioxidants in a mixture of antioxidants can be used in the treatment of cancer, thereby avoiding the possibility of toxicity at higher doses or of growth stimulation at lower doses of single antioxidants.

A mixture of antioxidants at low doses (vitamin A, 3.5 IU/day; vitamin E, 0.107 IU/day; and vitamin C, 4 mg/day) protected mice against damage to bone marrow caused by radioimmunotherapy (a treatment using antibodies containing strong radioactive substances) without affecting the growth of tumor cells. This is a very important observation in an animal tumor model, because it suggests that radiation oncologists' fear that these antioxidants can protect cancer cells is not justified.

A preliminary clinical study of human small-cell lung carcinoma suggests that the administration of high-dose multiple antioxidants (vitamin C in the form of ascorbic acid, 6,100 mg/day; natural α-tocopherol, 1,050 mg/day; and synthetic β-carotene, 60 mg/day) heightened the efficacy of standard therapy (carboplatin and paclitaxel, a form of taxol) by enhancing tumor response without reducing the objective toxicity to normal cells. Nonetheless, patients receiving both chemotherapy and antioxidants completed full cycles of chemotherapeutic agents. A further study using larger number of patients is needed to confirm these results.

Based on the laboratory data (cancer cells in culture and animal tumors) and very limited human studies, we have proposed a hypothesis that high-dose multiple micronutrients including antioxidants, B vitamins, and appropriate minerals, together with modifications in diet and lifestyle, may improve the efficacy of standard therapy by intensifying tumor response and limiting toxicity. This hypothesis is applicable to both adult and pediatric tumors, and it is being tested in humans. The specific nutritional protocol to be used as an adjunct to standard therapy in the treatment of adult cancer is described here:

1. A multiple micronutrient preparation containing both β-carotene and vitamin A, two forms of vitamin E (*d*-α-tocopheryl succinate and *d*-α-tocopherol), vitamin C (calcium ascorbate), vitamin D, B vitamins, and appropriate minerals without iron, copper, or manganese (a preparation available commercially from Scientific Nutrition).

2. An additional 8 g of vitamin C in the form of calcium ascorbate, 800 IU of *d*-α-tocopheryl succinate, and 60 mg of natural β-carotene, divided into two doses— half in the morning and half in the evening before meals.

3. A diet low in fat (no more than 10 percent of calories from fat) and high in fiber (26 g/day from fruits and vegetables and fiber-supplemented cereals) and avoidance of nitrite-rich meat, such as bacon, sausage, and deli meats. Cancer patients, however, may not tolerate the recommended amounts of fiber during the course of therapy.

4. A lifestyle of limited stress, no smoking, no excess consumption of caffeine-containing beverages or alcoholic beverages, and regular moderate exercise (three to four times per week).

The specific micronutrient protocol to be used in combination with standard therapy in the treatment of childhood cancer is the following:

1. A multiple micronutrient preparation containing both β-carotene and vitamin A, two forms of vitamin E (*d*-α-tocopheryl succinate and *d*-α-tocopherol), vitamin C (calcium ascorbate), vitamin D, B vitamins, and appropriate minerals without iron, copper, or manganese (a preparation

available commercially from Scientific Nutrition in Oakland, California).

2. An additional 2 g of vitamin C in the form of calcium ascorbate, 200 IU of d-α-tocopheryl succinate, and 15 mg of natural β-carotene, divided into two doses, half in the morning and half in the evening before meals.

3. A diet low in fat and high in fiber and avoidance of nitrite-rich meat, such as bacon, sausage, and deli meats. In children less than five years of age, the proposed diet may not be applicable in totality. Efforts should be made, however, to feed fruit and vegetable preparations and juices made from grapes, oranges, and carrots.

4. A lifestyle of limited stress, no smoking (teenagers), no excess consumption of caffeine-containing beverages or any consumption of alcoholic beverages (teenagers), and regular moderate exercise (three to four times per week). Some of these guidelines may not be applicable to a child less than five years of age, but every effort should be made to lessen the physical and emotional stress of the child.

This protocol should be started 48 hours before standard therapy and continued for the entire period of treatment. After the completion of treatment, both adults and children should take a multiple micronutrient preparation as before; however, the additional antioxidant doses should be reduced gradually (over a period of several months) by half. Diet and lifestyle modifications for children remain the same until they are sixteen years of age, after which the protocol for high-risk adult populations should be adopted (see chapter 6). This maintenance micronutrient protocol should be followed throughout the person's life.

In contrast to the hypothesis proposed by us, there is another theory that antioxidants protect cancer cells against damage produced by X-irradiation and chemotherapeutic agents and therefore should not be used in combination with standard therapy in cancer treatment. This hypothesis is based on theoretical assumptions that are not supported by experimental data, and speculative extrapolation of data that were obtained without the use of radiation or chemotherapeutic agents. One of the assumptions is that since antioxidants destroy free radicals, and since they protect normal cells against damage produced by free radicals, they must also protect cancer cells against such damage. Experimental data published on cells in culture and animal tumor models with high-dose vitamin A, C, and E, and β-carotene support the first assumption regarding normal cells but do not bear out the second part of the assumption regarding cancer cells. As a matter of fact, these antioxidants amplify the effects of X-irradiation and chemotherapeutic agents on tumor cells.

In another study, it was noted that following administration of radioactive ascorbic acid, vitamin C accumulated in tumor cells more than in the brain. This finding was interpreted to mean that vitamin C will protect cancer cells against damage produced by irradiation and chemotherapeutic agents, but this study did not use radiation or any chemotherapeutic agent. There are no direct experimental data on high-dose vitamin C and cancer cells that endorse this hypothesis. As a matter of fact, there are substantial data that show that high-dose vitamin C enhances the effects of irradiation and chemotherapeutic agents on tumor cells but protects normal cells against the adverse effects of these agents.

In one study, a group of genetically engineered mice (transgenic mice) who had a high incidence of spontaneous tumors were used to study the effects of vitamin A and E deficiency on tumor growth. The group of animals, who were made 90 percent deficient in vitamin A and E, showed a reduced rate of growth of tumors compared with those that were not deficient in these antioxidants. This is not surprising, because cancer cells (like normal cells) require small amounts of antioxidants for growth. Investigators, however, interpreted their results to mean that high-dose antioxidants protect cancer cells against the damaging effects of irradiation and chemotherapeutic agents. Again, no X-irradiation or any chemotherapeutic agent was used in this study. In humans, vitamin A deficiency will cause night blindness, and vitamin E deficiency will cause irreversible neurological damage. Therefore, such studies have no relevance in the treatment of human cancer. As a matter of fact, a wild extrapolation of data creates unnecessary confusion among health professionals.

A large clinical trial to assess the role of high-dose micronutrients, including multiple antioxidants in combination with standard therapy, is being planned by the Cancer Treatment Center of America. Another trial is in progress at the Henry Ford Hospital in Detroit and at the All India Medical Institute in New Delhi. It is hoped that these studies will provide conclusive evidence concerning whether high-dose multiple antioxidants can improve the efficacy of standard therapy in the treatment of human cancer.

Designing a Nutrition and Lifestyle Program for Those Who Are in Remission after Standard Therapy

The current standard therapy has produced a growing number of cancer patients in remission, but these patients still face the risk of recurring cancer, the development of new tumors induced by treatment agents, and the risk of noncancerous diseases. It would be a major contribution to the efficacy of standard treatment if any of these risks could be reduced through the use of micronutrient supplements.

What Is Remission and How Is It Achieved?

During remission, cancer cannot be detected by known technologies, either because there are very few cancer cells left or because there are no cancer cells at all. Surgery, extensive chemotherapy, and radiation therapy can bring about a remission in certain types of tumors, if they are detected at early stages. These types include neuroblastoma, Wilms tumor, Hodgkin disease, certain childhood leukemias, breast cancer, cervical cancer, prostate cancer, and melanoma.

What Are the Consequences of Standard Cancer Therapies?

There are four possible major consequences of cancer treatment:

1. The person becomes free of cancer.

2. The original cancer can recur, generally within five to ten years, because a few cancer cells were left after treatment and they could not be eliminated by the body's defense system.

3. The person may be cured of the original cancer, but new tumors may develop ten to thirty years after treatment.

4. Noncancerous diseases and adverse effects may develop, such as paralysis, reproductive failure, reduction in growth, aplastic anemia, cataracts, or necrosis of several vital organs (brain, liver, muscle, etc.).

Some laboratory experiments suggest that we can influence some of the factors leading to recurrence and adverse effects by designing an appropriate diet, together with appropriate amounts of supplemental micronutrients such as those given after the completion of standard therapy. Dietary and lifestyle guidelines such as those described for the prevention of cancer in high-risk populations (chapter 5) should be followed. It should be emphasized that the efficacy of the proposed nutritional protocol has not been tested in humans.

What Results Might Be Expected from Adhering to a Proper Diet and Taking Supplemental Micronutrients?

The proper diet and micronutrient supplementation might stop or postpone cancer recurrence, prevent or delay the onset of new cancer, or avert or delay the onset of a noncancerous disease or the various side effects of therapy. We must emphasize that our suggestions regarding diet, supplemental vitamins, and lifestyle are based only on animal studies, some human studies, and the known safe limits of the nutrients.

Concluding Remarks

The efficacy of standard therapy, which includes surgery, radiation therapy, and chemotherapy, has reached a plateau for many cancers. In cases where remission or cure of a cancer has been achieved, there are risks of recurrence of the original tumor, the development of new tumors induced by treatment agents, and the appearance of noncancerous diseases among cancer survivors. We have proposed a nutritional protocol and modifications in diet and lifestyle, in combination with standard therapy, that may heighten tumor response to standard therapeutic agents and minimize toxicities during treatment of both adult and childhood cancers. Extensive laboratory data and some limited human studies support our hypothesis.

A contradicting hypothesis has proposed that antioxidants actually protect cancer cells against the damaging effects of X-irradiation and chemotherapeutic agents. This rationale is based on theoretical assumptions and extrapolation of the results of studies in which no radiation or chemotherapeutic agents were used. We also have recommended that whenever heat therapy is used, it must be in the form of whole-body treatment at low temperatures (40–41°C). The patient should take the nutritional supplements advocated for cancer treatment before any standard therapy is initiated.

7 Recommended Dietary Allowances

Definition of Recommended Dietary Allowances

Recommended dietary allowances (RDAs) are defined as the levels of intake of essential nutrients that, on the basis of scientific knowledge, are judged by the Food and Nutrition Board to be adequate to meet the known nutrient needs of practically all healthy persons. It has been stated clearly that RDAs are neither minimal requirements nor optimal levels of intake.

Relationship Between Recommended Dietary Allowances and Health

Unlike the laboratory rodent diet, human diets are diverse and contain substances that have opposing influences on the process of carcinogenesis. The levels of each of these cancer-protective and cancer-causing agents in the diet vary from one person to another and from one time to another, even on the same day in the same person. The susceptibility of different people to these agents differs depending upon genetic, environmental, and lifestyle-related factors. Some potential mutagens and carcinogens occur naturally in the diet, some are formed during cooking, and some are generated during digestion. Thus, the gastrointestinal tract is a major site of important biological reactions that produce mutagens and carcinogens. The levels of these toxins, which are dependent upon the type of food eaten, can be considered a major determinant of the risk of cancer and other diseases.

In view of these complexities, it is not possible to determine the levels of nutrients needed for optimal health or disease prevention. This difficulty has been acknowledged in the tenth edition of the National Academy of Sciences Recommended Dietary Allowances. Nevertheless, it is highly commendable that since 1941, a group of experts has developed RDA values for different nutrients. From time to time, these values have been revised. There is no doubt that daily intake of RDA levels of nutrients prevents a deficiency and allows for normal growth and development, at least during the early phase of life. The fundamental question arises, "What are the levels of micronutrients for optimal health and disease prevention?" This is a debatable issue, and there is no uniformity of opinion among experts. There should not be any disagreement, however, on the fact that the incidence rates of various chronic illnesses, such as cancer, heart disease, and Alzheimer disease, are escalating in the midst of lengthening life spans.

Supplemental micronutrients, including antioxidants, have been useful in the prevention and treatment of some of these diseases. From these studies, we conclude that antioxidants at the RDA levels may not be sufficient for optimal health or disease prevention. For these reasons and others supported by the laboratory data, we suggest that supplementation with certain micronutrients at moderate doses (higher than RDAs), together with changes in diet and lifestyle-related factors, are essential. The guidelines proposed in chapters 5 and 6 for supplemental antioxidants, diet, and lifestyle have taken into consideration age and other risk factors, but their efficacy cannot be established until a well-controlled clinical trial in humans is performed, and the predicted efficacy is confirmed. Sample RDA values of nutrients have been listed in Tables 9 through 12. Energy, fat, and fiber contents of some foods are listed in Tables 13 through 15. These values should serve as useful guidelines for selecting types of food that may be valuable for health and disease prevention.

Table 9 — Recommended Dietary Allowances (RDA) for Vitamins

Vitamins	RDA/Day			
	Men	Women	Pregnant Women	Smokers
Vitamin A	3,300 IU	2,600 IU	2,600 IU	NA
Vitamin C	60 mg	60 mg	70 mg	100 mg
Vitamin E	10 IU	8 IU	10 IU	NA
Vitamin D	200 IU	200 IU	400 IU	NA
Vitamin K	80 mcg	80 mcg	NA	NA
Thiamine	1.22 mg	1.03 mg	1.53 mg	NA
Pantothenic Acid	4–7 mg (estimated)	4–7 mg (estimated)	NA	NA
Biotin	30–100 mcg	30–100 mcg	NA	NA
Riboflavin	1.2 mg	1.2 mg	1.5 mg	NA
Niacin	13 mg	13 mg	13 mg	NA
Vitamin B_6	2.0 mg	1.6 mg	2.2 mg	NA
Folate	200 mcg	180 mcg	400 mcg	NA
Vitamin B_{12}	2 mcg	2 mcg	2.2 mcg	NA

In the year 2000, the Institute of Medicine (a branch of the National Academy of Sciences) recommended raising the vitamin C daily intake from 60 mg to 90 mg for men and to 75 mg for women, with an extra 35 mg for smokers. The upper limit for vitamin C was set at 2,000 mg/day. The daily intake of vitamin E was increased from 8 mg for women and 10 mg for men to 15 mg for both, with an upper limit of 1,000 mg. The daily intake of selenium was raised from 55 mcg for women and 70 mcg for men to 55 mcg for both, with an upper limit of 400 mcg. The Food and Nutrition Board has not adopted these recommendations. Although the efforts of the Institute of Medicine to examine the current status of RDAs of certain nutrients must be applauded, a few problems associated with these recommendations must be pointed out. Nutrients other than vitamin C are depleted among smokers; therefore, it is not sufficient to raise only the values of vitamin C. The upper limits of vitamin E and selenium are high. The long-term consumption of such a large dose of vitamin E could induce defects in the blood-clotting mechanism. High doses of selenium could prompt cataract formation. Although the window of safety for vitamin E is very wide compared with its RDA value, this is not true for selenium.

Table 10 — Recommended Dietary Allowances (RDA) for Minerals

Minerals	RDA/Day			
	Men	Women	Pregnant Women	Postmenopausal Women
Calcium	800 mg	800 mg	1,200 mg	NA
Phosphorus	800 mg	800 mg	1,200 mg	NA
Magnesium	350 mg	280 mg	300 mg	NA

Table 11 — Recommended Dietary Allowances (RDAs) for Trace Metals

Trace Metals	RDA/Day			
	Men	Women	Pregnant Women	Postmenopausal Women
Iron	10 mg	15 mg	30 mg	10 mg
Zinc	15 mg	12 mg	15 mg	NA
Iodine	150 mcg	150 mcg	175 mcg	NA
Copper	1.5 mg	1.5 mg	NA	NA
Manganese	2.0–5 mg	2.0–5 mg	NA	NA
Fluoride	1.5–4 mg	1.5–4 mg	NA	NA
Chromium	50–200 mcg	50–200 mcg	NA	NA
Molybdenum	75–250 mcg	75–250 mcg	NA	NA
Selenium	70 mcg	55 mcg	NA	NA

Table 12 — Recommended Dietary Allowances (RDA) for Nutrients

Nutrients	RDA/Day
Carbohydrate	No specific requirements; 287 g for men, 117 g for women (estimated intake)
Fiber	No specific requirements; 12 g (estimated intake)
Protein	0.75 g per kilogram of body weight or 56.3 g for a 75-kilogram (165 pound) person (estimated intake)
Fat	No specific requirements; about 36.4% of total calories (estimated intake)
Calories	2,300–2,900 for men and 1,900–2,200 for women

Table 13 — Energy Content of Selected Foods

Food	Portion Size	Kcal/Portion
Meat	3 ounces	200–250
Egg	1 large	80
Shrimp	3 ounce	78
Tuna	3 ounces	78
Cheese	1 ounce	107–114
Ice Cream	1/2 cup	135
Milk, whole	1 cup	150
Milk, skim	1 cup	85
Yogurt, low fat	1 cup	140
Bread, whole wheat	1 slice	56
Rice, cooked	1/2 cup	100
Kidney beans, cooked	1/2 cup	110
Green beans, cooked	1/2 cup	18
Carrot	1 medium	34
Corn on the cob	5 1/2 inches	160
Peas	1/2 cup	86
Apple	1	80
Banana	1	100
Orange	1	65
Peach	1	38
Pear	1	100
Butter	1 tbsp	100
Peanuts	1 ounce	172
Potato chips	10 chips	115

Table 14 — Fat Content of Selected Foods

Food	Portion Size	Grams/Portion
Bacon, crisp	2 slices	6
Beef, roast	3 ounces	26
Chicken, baked—with skin	3 ounces	11
Chicken, baked—without skin	3 ounces	6
Egg, boiled	1	6
Pork chop	3 ounces	19
Shrimp	3 ounces	0.9
Tuna	3 ounces	0.9
Cheese, Cheddar	1 ounce	9
Ice cream	1/2 cup	7
Milk, whole	1 cup	8
Milk, skim	1 cup	1
Sour cream	1 tbsp	3
Yogurt, low fat	1 cup	4
Biscuit	1	4
Bread	1 slice	1
Cornbread	1 piece	7
Oatmeal, cooked	1/2 cup	1
Avocado	1/8	4
Margarine	1 tsp	4
Mayonnaise	1 tbsp	11
Peanut butter	1 tbsp	7
Vegetable oil	1 tsp	5

Table 15 — Fiber Content of Selected Foods

Food	Portion Size	Grams/Portion
Beef	0	0
Dairy products	0	0
All-bran cereal	1 cup	25.6
Bran muffin	1	4.2
Raisin bran cereal	1 cup	6
White bread	1 slice	0.8
Whole wheat bread	1 slice	1.3
Broccoli	1/2 cup	3.2
Carrot, raw	1 medium	2.4
Corn	1/2 cup	4.6
Apple, with skin	1	3
Pear, with skin	1	3.8
Raspberries	1/2 cup	4.6

Concluding Remarks

The RDA values are important guidelines for human health; however, for optimal health and disease prevention, moderate supplements of certain micronutrients, together with a balanced diet and changes in lifestyle, are essential. Conclusive human studies on this issue have not been conducted. Therefore, the efficacy of our proposed recommendations remains to be determined in humans.

Appendix:

Major Centers for Studies on Antioxidants, Diet, and Cancer

Studies on Cancer Treatment

Dr. Gerald M. Haase (cancer treatment), Rocky Mountain Medical Institute, Greenwood Village, CO 80121, U.S.A.

Dr. Jae Ho Kim (cancer treatment), Department of Radiation Oncology, Henry Ford Hospital, Detroit, MI 48202, U.S.A.

Dr. F. L. Meyskens, Jr. (treatment of human cancer, vitamin A), University of California Cancer Center, Orange, CA 92668, U.S.A.

Dr. G. E. Goodman (treatment of human cancer, vitamin A), Tumor Institute of Swedish Hospital, Seattle, WA 98104, U.S.A.

Dr. G. Mathé (treatment of human cancer, vitamin A), Service des Maladies Sanguines et Tumorales, Institut de Cancérologie et d'Immunogénétique (INSERM U-50), Hôpital Paul-Broussé, F-94804, France

Dr. G. J. S. Rustin (treatment of human cancer, vitamin A), Department of Medical Oncology, Charing Cross Hospital, London W68 RF, U.K.

Dr. W. J. Uphouse (treatment of human cancer, vitamin A), Cancer Center of Hawaii, Honolulu, HI 96813, U.S.A.

Dr. L. Itri (treatment of human cancer, vitamin A), Hoffmann–La Roche, Inc., Nutley, NJ 07110, U.S.A.

Dr. N. J. Lowe (treatment of human cancer, vitamin A), Division of Dermatology, School of Medicine, University of California at Los Angeles, Los Angeles, CA 90024, U.S.A.

Dr. M. M. Black (treatment of human cancer, vitamins A and E), Department of Pathology, New York Medical College, Valhalla, NY 10595, U.S.A.

Dr. Josef Beuth (cancer treatment), University of Cologne, Cologne, Germany

Dr. Keith I. Block (cancer treatment), Institute for Integrative Cancer Care, Evanston, IL, U.S.A.

Dr. W. L. Robinson (treatment of human cancer, vitamin A), Division of Oncology, Department of Medicine, University of Colorado Health Sciences Center, Denver, CO 80262, U.S.A.

Dr. G. L. Peck (treatment of human cancer, vitamin A), Dermatology Branch, National Cancer Institute, Bethesda, MD 20205, U.S.A.

Dr. W. Bollag and Dr. H. R. Hartmann (treatment of human cancer, vitamin A), Pharmaceutical Research Development, F. Hoffmann–La Roche & Co., Ltd., CH–4002, Basel, Switzerland

Dr. Balz Frei, Linus Pauling Institute, Oregon State University, Corvallis, OR 97331-6512, U.S.A.

Dr. F. Morishige (treatment of human cancer, vitamin C), Tachiarai Hospital, Fukuoka 838, Japan

Dr. Vinod Kochupillai (human cancer, β-carotene, and vitamin E), Department of Oncology, All India Institute of Medical Sciences, New Delhi, India

Dr R. T. Chlebowski (human cancer and vitamin K), School of Medicine, Harbor–UCLA Medical Center, Los Angeles, CA, U.S.A.

Dr. Abram Hoffer (human cancer and multiple vitamins), Hoffer Clinic, Victoria, British Columbia, Canada

Dr. Gian Maria Paganelli (vitamins), Istituto di Clinica Medica e Gastroenterologia, Policlinico S. Orsola, I-40138, Bologna, Italy

Dr. Scott Lippman (β-carotene retinoids), Department of Medical Oncology, University of Texas M. D. Anderson Cancer Center, Houston, TX 77030, U.S.A.

Dr. Charles B. Simone (cancer treatment), Simone Protective Cancer Center, Lawrenceville, N.J., U.S.A.

Studies on Human Cancer Prevention

Dr. T. Moon (vitamin A), Cancer Center, University of Arizona Health Sciences Center, Tucson, AZ 85724, U.S.A.

Dr. J. Li (vitamins A, C, and E), Department of Epidemiology and Cancer Institute, Chinese Academy of Medical Sciences, Beijing, People's Republic of China

Dr. L. M. De Luca, Dr. W. De Wys, and Dr. P. Greenwald (vitamins A, C, and E), National Cancer Institute, Bethesda, MD 20205, U.S.A.

Dr. C. Hennekens (vitamin A), Harvard Medical School, Boston, MA 02115, U.S.A.

Dr. R. L. Phillips (diets), Loma Linda Studies School of Health, Loma Linda University, Loma Linda, CA 92350, U.S.A.

Dr. C. Mettlin (vitamin A), Roswell Park Memorial Institute, Buffalo, NY 14263, U.S.A.

Dr. S. Graham (vitamin A), Departments of Sociology and Social and Preventive Medicine, State University of New York at Buffalo, Buffalo, NY 14214, U.S.A.

Dr. G. Kvale (vitamins A, C, and E), Institute of Hygiene and Social Medicine, University of Bergen, Bergen, Norway

Dr. M. Micksche (vitamin A), Institute of Cancer Research, University of Vienna, and Ludwig Boltzmann Institute for Clinical Oncology, Municipal Hospital, Lainz-Vienna, Austria

Dr. R. Doll (vitamins A, C, and E), Imperial Cancer Research Fund, Cancer Epidemiology Unit, Oxford, OX1 3QG, U.K.

Dr. R. Peto (vitamins A, C, and E), Department of Clinical Medicine, Imperial Cancer Research Fund Cancer Unit, Nuffield, Radcliffe Infirmary, Oxford, OX2 6HE, U.K.

Dr. Tim Buyers (antioxidants and diet), Department of Preventive Medicine, University of Colorado Health Sciences Center, Denver, CO 80262, U.S.A.

Dr. Dan Nixon (antioxidants and diet), American Health Foundation, New York, NY 10017, U.S.A.

Dr. J. Wylie-Rosett (vitamin A), Department of Community Health, Albert Einstein College of Medicine, Bronx, NY 10461, U.S.A.

Dr. A. J. Tuyns (vitamin C), Unit of Analytical Epidemiology, International Agency for Research on Cancer, F-69372, Lyon, Cedex 08, France

Dr. R. Burton (vitamins A, C, and E), Research Institute for Social Security, Helsinki, Finland

Dr. P. Helms (vitamins A, C, and E), Institute of Hygiene, Aarhus, Denmark

Dr. L. Bjerrum and Dr. A. Paerregaard (vitamins A, C, and E), Saint Elizabeth Hospital, Copenhagen, Denmark

Dr. J. H. Cummings and Dr. W. J. Branch (vitamins A, C, and E), Dunn Clinical Nutrition Center, Addenbrook's Hospital, Cambridge, U.K.

Dr. S. A. Broitman (alcohol and nutrition), Departments of Pathology and Microbiology, Boston University School of Medicine, Boston, MA 02118, U.S.A.

Dr. B. S. Reddy and Dr. J. H. Wisburger (fiber), Naylor Dana Institute for Disease Prevention, American Health Foundation, Valhalla, NY 10595, U.S.A.

Dr. T. Campbell (diets and nutrition), Division of Nutritional Sciences, Cornell University, Ithaca, NY 14850, U.S.A.

Dr. J. J. DeCosse (vitamins C and E), Department of Surgery, New York Hospital Cornell Medical Center, New York, NY 10021, U.S.A.

Dr. G. A. Kune (nutrition and cancer), Department of Surgery, University of Melbourne, Richmond 3121, Victoria, Australia

Dr. Shu-Yu (nutrition and cancer), Cancer Institute Chinese Academy of Medical Science, Beijing, People's Republic of China

Dr. A. Costa (retinoids and cancer), Istituto Nazionale Tumori, 20133 Milan, Italy

Dr. Leonida Santamaria (β-carotene and cancer), University of Pavia, Pavia, Italy

Michael J. Hill (nutrition and cancer), PHLS-CAMR, Salisbury, SP4 0JG, U.K.

Dr. G. H. McIntosh (nutrition and cancer), CSIRO Division of Human Nutrition, Adelaide, Australia

Dr. Paul Knekt (nutrition and cancer), Social Insurance Institution, SF-00381 Helsinki, Finland

Dr. C. E. Butterworth (folate and vitamin B_{12}), Department of Nutrition Science, University of Alabama at Birmingham, Birmingham, AL 35294, U.S.A.

Dr. H. S. Garewal (retinoid and β-carotene), Section of Hematology-Oncology, Tucson VA Medical Center, Tucson, AZ 85723, U.S.A.

Dr. Robert Bruce (vitamins), Ludwig Institute for Cancer Research, Toronto, Ontario, Canada

Dr. L. E. Holm (nutrition and cancer), Department of Cancer Prevention, Norrbacka, Karolinski Hospital, Stockholm, Sweden

Dr. E. C. Meyer (vitamin E), Department of Pharmacology, University of Pretoria, Pretoria, South Africa

Dr. E. B. Thorling (nutrition and cancer prevention), Danish Cancer Society, Department of Nutrition and Cancer, Norrebrograle 44 DK-8000, Denmark

Dr. N. V. Zandwick (nutrition and cancer prevention), Netherlands Cancer Institute, 1066 CX Amsterdam, Netherlands

Laboratory Studies

Dr. E. Seifter (vitamin A), Department of Surgery, Albert Einstein College of Medicine, Bronx, NY 10461, U.S.A.

Dr. R. C. Moon (vitamin A), Laboratory of Pathophysiology, IIT Research Institute, Chicago, IL 60616, U.S.A.

Dr. T. K. Basu (vitamins A and C), Department of Food and Nutrition, University of Alberta, Edmonton, Alberta T6G2M8, Canada

Dr. L. Santamaria (vitamin A and β-carotene), C. Department of Pharmacology, University of Pavia, I-27100 Pavia, Italy

Dr. N. T. Telang (vitamins), Laboratory of Molecular Biology and Virology, Memorial Sloan-Kettering Cancer Center, New York, NY 10021, U.S.A.

Dr. S. Takase (vitamins), Departments of Nutrition and Biochemistry, Shizuoka Women's University, Shizuoka-City, Shizuoka 422, Japan

Dr. T. J. Slaga (vitamins A, C, and E), American Medical Center, Denver, CO 80262, U.S.A.

Dr. P. Newberne (vitamin E and selenium), Massachusetts Institute of Technology, Cambridge, MA 02139, U.S.A.

Dr. K. N. Prasad (vitamins E and C), Department of Radiology, Center for Vitamin and Cancer Research, University of Colorado Health Sciences Center, Denver, CO 80262, U.S.A.

Dr. E. Bright-See (vitamins E and C), and Dr. H. Newmark (vitamins), Ludwig Institute for Cancer Research, Toronto, Ontario, M4Y1M4, Canada

Dr. R. P. Tengerdy (vitamin E), Department of Microbiology, Colorado State University, Fort Collins, CO 80523, U.S.A.

Dr. S. V. Kandarkar (vitamin A), Cancer Research Institute, Parel Bombay, India

Dr. D. G. Hendricks (vitamins), Departments of Nutrition and Food Sciences, Utah State University, Logan, UT 84322, U.S.A.

Dr. R. Lotan (vitamin A), Department of Tumor Biology, M.D. Anderson Hospital and Tumor Institute, Houston, TX 77030, U.S.A.

Dr. Y. M. Yang (vitamin E), M. D. Anderson Hospital and Tumor Institute, University of Texas System Cancer Center, Houston, TX 77030, U.S.A.

Dr. L. W. Wattenberg (vitamin E and other antioxidants), Department of Pathology, University of Minnesota, Minneapolis, MN 55455, U.SA.

Dr. B. P. Sani (vitamin C), Kettering Meyer Laboratory, Southern Research Institute, Birmingham AL 35203, U.S.A.

Dr. A. M. Jetten (vitamin A), National Institute of Environmental Health Sciences, Research Triangle, NC 27709, U.S.A.

Dr. E. P. Norkus (vitamin C), Dr. H. Bhagavan (vitamins A, C, and E) and Dr. L. Machlin (vitamin E), Hoffmann–LaRoche, Inc., Nutley, NJ 07110, U.S.A.

Dr. R. Gol-Winkler (vitamin C), Laboratoire de Chimie Médicale, Institut de Pathologie, Université de Liège, B-4000, Start Tilman Liège 1, Belgium

Dr. H. C. Park (vitamin C), Department of Medicine, University of Kansas Medical Center, Kansas City, KS 66103, U.S.A.

Dr. B. P. Sethi (vitamin C), Oncology Research Center, Bowman Gray School of Medicine of Wake Forest University, Winston-Salem, NC 27103, U.S.A.

Dr. J. A. Eisman (vitamins), University of Melbourne, Respiratory General Hospital, Heidelberg 3084, Victoria, Australia

Dr. M. Hozumi (vitamins A and E), Department of Chemotherapy, Saitama Cancer Center, Research Unit, Saitama 362, Japan

Dr. L. H. Chen (vitamins C and E), Department of Nutrition and Food Services, University of Kentucky, Lexington, KY 40506, U.S.A.

Dr. H. Fortmeyer (vitamins), Tieversuchsanlage des Klinikum der J.W. Goethe-universität, D-6000, Frankfurt, Germany

Dr. M. B. Sporn (vitamin A), Laboratory of Chemoprevention, National Cancer Institute, Bethesda, MD 20892, U.S.A.

Dr. F. Chytil (vitamin A), Departments of Biochemistry and Medicine, Vanderbilt University, School of Medicine, Nashville, TN 37240, U.S.A.

Dr. A.T. Diplock (vitamin E and selenium), Department of Biochemistry, Royal Free Hospital, School of Medicine, University of London, London, U.K.

Dr. A. Trichopoulou (vitamins), Departments of Nutrition and Biochemistry, Athens School of Hygiene, GR-11521 Athens, Greece

Dr. G. N. Schrauzer (selenium), Department of Chemistry, University of California at San Diego, La Jolla, CA 92093, U.S.A.

Dr. J. W. Thanassi (vitamin B_{12}), Department of Biochemistry, College of Medicine, University of Vermont, Burlington, VT 05405, U.S.A.

Dr. G. P. Tryfiates (vitamin B_{12}), Department of Biochemistry, School of Medicine, West Virginia University, Morgantown, WV 26506, U.S.A.

Dr. D. G. Zaridze (vitamins), World Health Organization, Centre International de Recherche sur le Cancer, 69732 Lyon, Cedex 08, France

Dr. M. H. Zile (vitamins), Departments of Food Sciences and Human Nutrition, Michigan State University, East Lansing, MI 48824, U.S.A.

Dr. H. Fujuki (vitamins) and Dr. T. Sugimura (vitamins), National Cancer Center Research Institute, Tokyo 104, Japan

Dr. A. E. Rogers (vitamins), Departments of Nutrition and Food Sciences, Massachusetts Institute of Technology, Cambridge, MA 02139, U.S.A.

Dr. T. R. Breitmann (vitamins), National Cancer Institute, Bethesda, MD 20205, U.S.A.

Dr. P. B. McCay (vitamin E and antioxidants), Oklahoma Medical Foundation, Oklahoma City, OK 73104, U.S.A.

Dr. J. C. Bertram (vitamins), Grace Cancer Drug Center, Roswell Park Memorial Institute, Buffalo, NY 14263, U.S.A.

Dr. F. E. Jones (vitamin A), Department of Surgery, College of Medicine, Milwaukee, WI 53226, U.S.A.

Dr. B. S. Alam (vitamin A), Department of Biochemistry, Louisiana State University Medical Center, New Orleans, LA 70119, U.S.A.

Dr. G. Shklar (vitamin E), Departments of Oral Medicine and Oral Pathology, Harvard School of Dental Medicine, Boston, MA 02115, U.S.A.

Dr. D. M. Klurfeld (vitamin A), Wistar Institute of Anatomy and Biology, Philadelphia, PA 19104, U.S.A.

Dr. S. J. Van Rensburg (vitamin A), National Research Institute for Nutritional Diseases, Tygerberg, 7505 South Africa

Dr. D. M. Disorbo (vitamin B_6), Oncology Research Laboratory, Nassau Hospital, Mineola, NY 11501, U.S.A.

Dr. Y. Tomita (vitamin A), Department of Public Health, Kurume University School of Medicine, Kurume-830, Japan

Dr. A. R. Kennedy (protease inhibitors and antioxidants), Department of Radiation Oncology, University of Pennsylvania Medical School, Philadelphia, PA 19104, U.S.A.

Dr. K. K. Carroll (fat), Department of Biochemistry, University of Western Ontario, London, Ontario, N6A 5C1, Canada

Dr. B. N. Ames (diets and vitamins), Department of Biochemistry, University of California, Berkeley, CA 94720, U.S.A.

Dr. I. Emerit (antioxidants), Université de Pierre et Marie Curie, Paris, France

Dr. D. Schmahl (vitamin C), Institute of Toxicology and Chemotherapy, German Cancer Research Center, Heidelberg, Germany

Dr. Y. S. Hong (vitamins A, C, and E), College of Medicine, Ewha Women's University, Seoul, South Korea

Dr. C. Ip (vitamin E and selenium), Department of Breast Surgery, Roswell Park Memorial Institute, Buffalo, NY 14263, U.S.A.

Dr. L. G. Isreals (vitamin K), Manitoba Institute of Cell Biology, University of Manitoba, Winnipeg, Manitoba, Canada

Dr. R. G. Ham (nutrients), Department of Molecular, Cellular, and Developmental Biology, University of Colorado, Boulder, CO 80309, U.S.A.

Dr. J. P. Berry (selenium), SC 27 Inserm, Laboratoire de Biophysique, Faculté de Médecine, 94010 Créteil, France

Dr. M. Sakaguchi (fat), Department of Surgery, Kansai Medical University, Osaka 570, Japan

Dr. S. M. Przybyszewski (vitamin E and other antioxidants), Department of Biochemistry, Institute of Hematology, 00-957 Warsaw, Poland

Dr. C. Beckman (vitamin E), Biology Department, Concordia University, Montreal, Quebec, Canada

Dr. M. Menkes and Dr. G. Comstock (vitamin E), Johns Hopkins Training Center for Public Health Research, Hagerstown, MD 21740, U.S.A.

Dr. J. T. Salomen (selenium and human cancer), Department of Community Health, Research Institute of Public Health, University of Kuopio, 70221 Kuopio-1, Finland

Dr. M. G. Le (alcohol and human cancer), Institute Gustave Roussy, Villejuif, France

Dr. J. A. Milner (selenium and animal cancer), Department of Food Science, Division of Nutritional Sciences, University of Illinois, Urbana, IL 61801, U.S.A.

Dr. A. A. Yunis (vitamin D), Department of Medicine, University of Miami School of Medicine, Miami, FL 033101, U.S.A.

Dr. M. Murakoshi (carotenoids), Oleochemistry Research Center Lion Corporation, Tokyo 132, Japan

Dr. H. Takada (vitamin E), Department of Surgery, Kansai Medical University, Moriguchi, Osaka 570, Japan

Dr. K. Kline (vitamin E), Division of Nutritional Sciences, GEA 117, University of Texas, Austin, TX 78712–1097, U.S.A.

Dr. W. A. Behrens (vitamin E), Bureau of Nutritional Sciences Food Directorate, Health Protection Branch, Health and Welfare, Ottowa, Ontario, Canada

Dr. Clinton J. Grubbs (vitamin A), Department of Nutrition Sciences, University of Alabama at Birmingham, Birmingham, AL 35294, U.S.A.

Dr. A. Verma (retinoids), University of Wisconsin Clinical Cancer Center, Madison, WI 53792, U.S.A.

Dr. Maryce M. Jacobs (nutrition and cancer), American Institute for Cancer Research, Washington, D.C., 20009, U.S.A.

Dr. J. L. Schwartz (vitamins A and E), Howard Medical School, Washington, D.C., U.S.A.

Dr. Zulema Coppes, Faculty of Chemistry, University of Montevideo, Montevideo, Uruguay

Dr. William C. Cole, Department of Radiology, University of Colorado Health Sciences Center, Denver, Colorado, 80262, U.S.A.

Dr. K. L. Khanduja, Department of Biophysics, Postgraduate Institute of Medical Education and Research, Chandigarh, India

Further Reading

Ames, B. N. "Dietary Carcinogens and Anticarcinogens." *Science* 221 (1983): 1256–1264.

Barone, J., E. Taioli, J. R. Hebert, et al. "Vitamin Supplement Use and Risk of Oral and Esophageal Cancer." *Nutrition and Cancer* 18 (1992): 31–41.

Behrens, W. A., and R. Madere. "Tissue Discrimination Between RRR-α- and All-rac-α-tocopherols in Rats." *Journal of Nutrition* 121 (1991): 454–459.

Bendich, A., and J. A. Olson. "Biological Actions of Carotenoids." *Federation of American Society for Experimental Biology Journal* 3 (1989): 1927–1932.

Benedict, W. F., W. L. Wheatley, and P. A. Jones. "Inhibition of Chemically Induced Morphological Transformation and Reversion of the Transformed Phenotype by Ascorbic Acid in C3H/10T1/2 Cells." *Cancer Research* 40 (1980): 2796–2801.

Bianchi-Santamaria, A., S. Fedeli, and L. Santamaria. "Possible Activity of β-carotene in Patients with the AIDS-related Complex: A Pilot Study." *Medical Oncology and Tumor Pharmatherapeutics* 9 (1992): 151–153.

Bjelke, E. "Dietary Vitamin A and Human Lung Cancer." *International Journal of Cancer* 15 (1975): 562–565.

Black, M. M., R. E. Zachrau, A. S. Dion, et al. "Stimulation of Prognostically Favorable Cell-mediated Immunity of Breast Cancer Patients by High Dose Vitamin A and Vitamin E." In *Vitamins, Nutrition and Cancer,* edited by K. N. Prasad. Basel: Karger, 1984.

Blot, J., J.-Y. Li, P. R. Taylor, et al. "Nutrition Intervention Trials in Linxian, China: Supplementation with Specific Vitamins/Mineral Combinations, Cancer Incidence and Disease-specific Mortality in the General Population." *Journal of the National Cancer Institute* 85 (1993): 1483–1492.

Boutwell, R. K. "Biology and Biochemistry of the Two-step Model of Carcinogenesis." In *Modulation and Mediation of Cancer by Vitamins,* edited by F. L. Meyskens, Jr., and K. N. Prasad. Basel: Karger, 1983.

Broitman, S. A. "Relationship of Ethanolic Beverages and Ethanol to Cancers of the Digestive Tract." In *Vitamins, Nutrition and Cancer,* edited by K. N. Prasad. Basel: Karger, 1984.

Cadenas, E., and L. Packer. *Handbook of Antioxidants.* New York: Marcel Dekker, 1996.

Cameron, E., and L. Pauling. *Vitamin C and Cancer.* New York: Warner Books, 1981.

Carini, R., G. Poli, V. M. Dianzani, et al. "Comparative Evaluation of the Antioxidant Activity of α-Tocopherol, α-Tocopherol Polyethylene Glycol 1000 Succinate and α-Tocopheryl Succinate in Isolated Hepatocytes and Liver Microsomal Suspensions." *Biochemical Pharmacology* 39 (1990): 1597–1601.

Chow, C. K., R. R. Thacker, C. Changchit, et al. "Lower Levels of Vitamin C and Carotenes in Plasma of Cigarette Smokers." *Journal of the American College of Nutrition* 5 (1986): 305–312.

Cohrs, R. J., S. Torelli, K. N. Prasad, et al. "Effect of Vitamin E Succinate and cAMP-stimulating Agent on the Expression of c-*myc*, N-*myc* and H-*ras* in Murine Neuroblastoma Cells." *International Journal of Developmental Neuroscience* 9 (1991): 187–194.

Cole, W. C., and K. N. Prasad. "Contrasting Effects of Vitamins as Modulators of Apoptosis in Cancer Cells and Normal Cells: A Review." *Nutrition and Cancer* 29 (1997): 97–103.

Cole, P., and W. Sateren. "The Evolving Picture of Cancer in America." *Journal of the National Cancer Institute* 87 (1996): 159–160.

Cook, M. G., and P. McNamara. "Effect of Dietary Vitamin E on Dimethylhydrazine-induced Colonic Tumor in Mice." *Cancer Research* 40 (1980): 1329–1331.

DeCosse, J. J., H. H. Miller, and M. L. Lesser. "Effect of Wheat Fiber and Vitamins C and E on Rectal Polyps in Patients with Familial Adenomatous Polyposis." *Journal of the National Cancer Institute* 81 (1989): 1290–1297.

Diet, Nutrition and Cancer. Washington, D.C.: National Academy of Sciences Press, 1982.

Disorbo, D. M., and L. Nathanson. "High Dose Pyridoxal Supplemented Culture Medium Inhibits the Growth of a Human Malignant Melanoma Cell Line." *Nutrition and Cancer* 5 (1983): 10–15.

Doll, R., and R. Peto. "The Cause of Cancer: Quantitative Estimates of Available Risks of Cancer in the United States Today." *Journal of the National Cancer Institute* 66 (1981): 1192–1308.

Duthie, G. G., and J. R. Arthur. "Vitamin E Supplementation of Smokers and Non-smokers." *Fat Science and Technology* 11 (1990): 456–458.

Eicholzer, M., H. B. Stahelin, E. Ludin, and F. Bernasconi. "Plasma Vitamin C, E, Retinol and Carotene and Fatal Prostate Cancer: Seventeen-year Follow-up of the Prospective Basel Study." *Prostate* 38 (1999): 189–198.

Flavin, D. F., and A. C. Kolbye, Jr. "Nutritional Factors with a Potential to Inhibit Critical Pathways of Tumor Promotion." In *Modulation and Mediation of Cancer by Vitamins,* edited by F. L. Meyskens, Jr., and K. N. Prasad. Basel: Karger, 1983.

Fujiki, H., M. Suganuma, S. Okabe, et al. "Cancer Inhibition by Green Tea." *Mutation Research* 402 (1998): 307–310.

Furukawa, F., A. Nishikawa, K. I. Kasahara, I. S. Lee, K. Wakabayashi, M. Takahashi, and M. Hirose. "Inhibition by β-carotene of Upper Respiratory Tumorigenesis in Hamsters Receiving Diethyl Nitrosamine Followed by Cigarette Exposure." *Japanese Journal of Cancer Research* 90 (1999): 154–161.

Garewal, H. S., and F. L. Meyskens, Jr. "Retinoids and Carotenoids in the Prevention of Oral Cancer: A Critical Appraisal." *Cancer Epidemiology, Biomarkers and Prevention* 1 (1992): 155–159.

Geetha, A., R. Sankar, T. Mara, et al. "Alpha-Tocopherol Reduces Doxorubicin-induced Toxicity in Rats: Histological and Biochemical Evidence." *Indian Journal of Physiology and Pharmacology* 34 (1990): 94–100.

Gogn, S. R., J. L. Lertora, W. J. George, et al. "Protection of Zidovudine-induced Toxicity Against Murine Erythroid Progenitor Cells by Vitamin E." *Experimental Hematology* 19 (1991): 649–652.

Graham, S., C. Mettlin, J. Marshall, et al. "Dietary Factors in the Epidemiology of Cancer of the Larynx." *American Journal of Epidemiology* 113 (1981): 675–680.

Griffin, A. C. "Role of Selenium in the Chemoprevention of Cancer." *Advances in Cancer Research* 29 (1979): 419–442.

Gutterdge, J. M. C., and B. Halliwell. *Antioxidants in Nutrition, Health and Disease.* Oxford, England: Oxford University Press, 1994.

Haffke, S. C., and N. W. Seeds. "Neuroblastoma: The E. Coli of Neurobiology." *Life Sciences* 16 (1975): 1649–1658.

Hazuka, M. B., J. Edwards-Prasad, F. Newman, et al. "Beta-carotene Induces Morphological Differentiation and Decreases Adenylate Cyclase Activity in Melanoma Cells in Culture." *Journal of the American College of Nutrition* 9 (1990): 143–144.

Heimburger, D. C., B. Alexander, R. Birch, et al. "Improvement in Bronchial Squamous Metaplasia in Smokers Treated with Folate and Vitamin B_{12}." *Journal of the American Medical Association* 259 (1988): 1525–1530.

Higginson, J., and C. S. Muir. "Environmental Carcinogenesis: Misconceptions and Limitations to Cancer Control." *Journal of the National Cancer Institute* 63 (1979): 1291–1298.

Holm, L. E., E. Nordevang, M. L. Hjalmar, et al. "Treatment Failure and Dietary Habits in Women with Breast Cancer." *Journal of the National Cancer Institute* 85 (1993): 32–36.

Hong, W. K., S. M. Lippman, L. M. Itri, et al. "Prevention of Second Primary Tumors with Isotretinoin in Squamous-Cell Carcinoma of the Head and Neck." *New England Journal of Medicine* 323 (1990): 795–801.

Imashuku, S., T. Sugano, K. Fukiwara, et al. "Intra-aortic Prostaglandin E_1 (PGE_1) Infusion, Papaverine and Multiagent Chemotherapy in Disseminated Neuroblastoma." *Cancer Research* 23 (1983): 478a.

Imashuku, S., S. Todo, T. Amano, et al. "Cyclic AMP in Neuroblastoma, Ganglioneuroma and Sympathetic Ganglia." *Experientia* 33 (1977): 1507.

Ingold, K. U., G. W. Burton, D. O. Foster, et al. "Biokinetics of and Discrimination Between Dietary RRR- and SRR-α-tocopherols in the Male Rat." *Lipids* 22 (1987): 163–172.

Jain, M., G. M. Cook, F. G. Davis, et al. "A Case Control Study of Diet and Colorectal Cancer." *International Journal of Cancer* 26 (1980): 757–768.

Jiminez, J. J., and A. A. Yunis. "Protection from Chemotherapy-induced Alopecia by 1,2-Dimethylhydroxy Vitamin D_3." *Cancer Research* 52 (1992): 5123–5125.

Jones, F. E., R. A. Komorowski, and R. E. Condon. "The Effects of Ascorbic Acid and Butylated Hydroxyanisole in the Chemoprevention of 1,2-Dimethylhydrazine-induced Large Bowel Neoplasm." *Journal of Surgical Oncology* 25 (1984): 54–60.

Kennedy, A. R. "Prevention of Radiation Transformation In Vitro." In *Vitamins, Nutrition and Cancer,* edited by K. N. Prasad. Basel: Karger, 1984.

Khan, M. A., K. G. Jenkins, W. H. Tolleson, et al. "Retinoic Acid Inhibition of Human Papilloma Virus Type 16–mediated Transformation of Human Keratinocytes." *Cancer Research* 53: 905–909.

Kinlen, L. J., and K. McPherson. "Pancreas Cancer and Coffee and Tea Consumption: A Case-Control Study." *British Journal of Cancer* 49 (1984): 93–96.

Klurfeld, D. M., E. Aglow, S. A. Tepper, et al. "Modification of Dimethyl-hydrazine-induced Carcinogenesis in Rats by Dietary Cholesterol." *Nutrition and Cancer* 5 (1983): 16–23.

Knekt, P. "Role of Vitamin E in the Prophylaxis of Cancer." *Annals of Medicine* 23 (1991): 3–12.

Kritchevsky, D. "Diet and Nutrition Research." *Cancer* 62 (1988): 1839–1843.

Kummet, T., T. E. Moon, and F. L. Meyskens, Jr. "Vitamin A: Evidence for Its Preventive Role in Human Cancer." *Nutrition and Cancer* 5 (1983): 96–106.

Kune, G. A., and L. Vitetta. "Alcohol Consumption and the Etiology of Colorectal Cancer: A Review of Scientific Evidence from 1957 to 1991." *Nutrition and Cancer* 18 (1992): 97–111.

Kurek, M. P., and L. M. Corwin. "Vitamin E Protection Against Tumor Formation by Transplanted Murine Sarcoma Cells." *Nutrition and Cancer* 4 (1982): 128–139.

Labriola, D., and R. Livingston. "Possible Interactions Between Dietary Antioxidants and Chemotherapy." *Oncology* 13 (1999): 1003–1008.

Lambooy, J. P. "Influence of Riboflavin Antagonists on Azodye Hepatoma Induction in the Rat." *Proceedings of the Society for Experimental Biology and Medicine* 153 (1976): 532–535.

Lapre, J. A., H. T. De Vries, J. H. Koeman, et al. "The Antiproliferative Effect of Dietary Calcium on Colonic Epithelium Is Mediated by Luminal Surfactants and Dependent on the Type of Dietary Fat." *Cancer Research* 53 (1993): 784–789.

Le, M. G., C. Hill, A. Kramar, et al. "Alcoholic Beverage Consumption and Breast Cancer in a French Case-Control Study." *American Journal of Epidemiology* 120 (1984): 350–357.

Lippman, S. M., and F. L. Meyskens, Jr. "Vitamin A Derivatives in the Prevention and Treatment of Human Cancer." *Journal of the American College of Nutrition* 7 (1988): 269–284.

Lotan, R. "Effect of Vitamin A and Its Analogs (Retinoids) on Normal and Neoplastic Cells." *Biophysica Acta* 605 (1981): 33–91.

Menkes, M., and G. Comstock. "Vitamin A and E and Lung Cancer" [Abstract]. *American Journal of Epidemiology* 120 (1984): 491.

Meyskens, F. L., Jr. "Prevention and Treatment of Cancer with Vitamin A and Retinoids." In *Vitamins, Nutrition and Cancer,* edited by K. N. Prasad. Basel: Karger, 1984.

Meyskens, F. L., Jr., and K. N. Prasad, eds. *Modulation and Mediation of Cancer* by Vitamins. Basel: Karger, 1983.

Mihich, E., F. Rosen, and C. A. Nichol. "The Effect of Pyridoxine Deficiency on a Spectrum of Mouse and Rat Tumors." *Cancer Research* 19 (1959): 1244–1248.

Moss, R. W. *Antioxidants Against Cancer.* New York: Equinox Press, 2000.

Murakoshi, M., H. Nishino, Y. Satomi, et al. "Potent Prevention Action of β-carotene Against Carcinogenesis: Spontaneous Liver Carcinogenesis and Promoting Stage of Lung and Skin Carcinogenesis in Mice Are Suppressed More Effectively by

Carotene Than by β-carotene." *Cancer Research* 52 (1992): 6583–6587.

Nakachi, K., K. Suemasu, K. Suga, T. Takeo, K. Imai, and Y. Higushi. "Influence of Drinking Green Tea on Breast Cancer Malignancy among Japanese Patients." *Japanese Journal of Cancer Research* 89 (1998): 254–261.

Newbern, P. M., and V. Suphakarn. "Nutrition and Cancer. A Review with Emphasis on the Role of Vitamin C, Vitamin E and Selenium." *Nutrition and Cancer* 5 (1983): 107–117.

Newmark, H. L., and M. Lipkin. "Colonic Hyperplasia and Hyperproliferation Induced in Rodents by a Nutritional Stress Diet Containing Four Factors of the Western Human Diet: High Fat and Phosphate, Low Calcium and Vitamin D." In *Calcium, Vitamin D and Prevention of Colon Cancer,* edited by M. Lipkin, H. L. Newmark, and G. Kelloff. Boca Raton, Fla.: CRC Press, 1991.

Novogrodsky, A., A. Dvir, T. Sholnik, et al. "Effect of Polar Organic Compounds on Leukemic Cells: Butyrate Induced Partial Remission of Acute Myelogenous Leukemia in a Child." *Cancer* 51 (1983): 9–11.

O'Dell, B. L., and R. A. Sande, eds. *Handbook of Nutritionally Essential Mineral Elements.* New York: Marcel Dekker, 1997.

Odukoya, O., F. Hawach, and G. Shaklar. "Retardation of Experimental Oral Cancer by Topical Vitamin E." *Nutrition and Cancer* 6 (1984): 98–104.

Ohkoshi, M., H. Ohta, and M. Ito. "Effect of Vitamin B_2 on Tumorigenesis of 3-Methylcholanthrene in the Mouse." Gan To Kagaku Ryoho (Japan) 73 (1982): 105–107.

Paganelli, G. M., G. Biasco, G. Brandi, et al. "Effect of Vitamins A, C and E Supplementation on Rectal Cell Proliferation in

Patients with Colorectal Adenomas." *Journal of the National Cancer Institute* 84 (1992): 47–51.

Palgi, A. "Vitamin A and Lung Cancer." *Nutrition and Cancer* 6 (1984): 105–119.

Prasad, K. N. "Differentiation of Neuroblastoma Cells in Culture." *Biological Reviews* 50 (1975): 129–165.

———. "Butyric Acid: A Small Fatty Acid with Diverse Biological Functions." *Life Sciences* 27 (1980): 1351–1358.

———. "Therapeutic Potentials of Differentiating Agents in Neuroblastomas." In *Biology of Cancer,* vol. 2, edited by E. A. Mirand, W. B. Hutchinson, and E. Mihich. New York: Alan R. Liss, 1983.

———, ed. *Vitamins, Nutrition and Cancer.* Basel: Karger, 1984.

———. "Induction of Differentiated Phenotypes in Melanoma Cells by a Combination of an Adenosine 3',5'-Cyclic Monophosphate Stimulating Agent and *d*-α-Tocopheryl Succinate." Cancer Letters 44 (1989): 17–22.

———. "Vitamin E and Cancer Prevention: Recent Advances and Future Potentials." *Journal of the American College of Nutrition* 11 (1992): 487–500.

———, R. J. Cohrs, and O. K. Sharma. "Decreased Expression of c-*myc* and H-*ras* Oncogenes in Vitamin E Succinate–induced Morphologically Differentiated Murine B-16 Melanoma Cells in Culture." *Biochemistry and Cell Biology* 68 (1990): 1250–1255.

———, W. Cole, and P. Hovland. "Cancer Prevention Studies: Past, Present and Future." *Nutrition* 14 (1998): 197–210.

———, W. C. Cole, and J. E. Prasad. "Multiple Antioxidant Vitamins as an Adjunct to Standard and Experimental Cancer Therapies." *Journal of Oncology* 31 (1999): 101–108.

————, and J. Edwards-Prasad. "Effect of Tocopherol (Vitamin E) Acid Succinate on Morphological Alteration and Growth Inhibition in Melanoma Cells in Culture." *Cancer Research* 43 (1982): 550–555.

————, A. Kumar, M. Kochupillai, and W. Cole. "High Doses of Multiple Antioxidant Vitamins: Essential Ingredients in Improving the Efficacy of Standard Cancer Therapy." *Journal of the American College of Nutrition* 18 (1999): 13–25.

————, and B. N. Rama. "Modification of the Effect of Pharmacological Agents on Tumor Cells in Culture by Vitamin C and Vitamin E." In *Modulation and Mediation of Cancer by Vitamins,* edited by F. L. Meyskens, Jr., and K. N. Prasad. Basel: Karger, 1983.

Recommended Dietary Allowances, tenth edition. Washington, D.C.: National Academy of Sciences, 1989.

Reddy, B. S. "Dietary Macronutrients and Colon Cancer." In *Vitamins, Nutrition and Cancer,* edited by K. N. Prasad. Basel: Karger, 1984.

Rimm, E. B., M. J. Stampfer, A. Ascherio, et al. "Vitamin E Consumption and the Risk of Coronary Disease in Men." *New England Journal of Medicine* 328 (1993): 1450–1456.

Risch, H.A., G. R. Howe, M. Jain, et al. "Are Female Smokers at Higher Risk for Lung Cancer Than Male Smokers? A Case-Control Analysis by Histologic Type." *American Journal of Epidemiology* 138 (1993): 281–293.

Rosenberg, R. N. "Neuroblastoma and Glioma Cell Cultures in Studies of Neurologic Functions: The Clinician's Rosetta Stone." *Neurology* 27 (1977): 105–108.

Sahu, S. N., J. Edwards-Prasad, and K. N. Prasad. "Effect of α-Tocopheryl Succinate on Adenylate Cyclase Activity in Murine Neuroblastoma Cells in Culture." *Journal of the American College of Nutrition* 7 (1988): 285–293.

Salonen, J. T., G. Alfthan, J. K. Huttunen, et al. "Association Between Serum Selenium and the Risk of Cancer." *American Journal of Epidemiology* 120 (1984): 342–349.

Schrauzer, G. N. "Selenium in Nutritional Cancer Prophylaxis: An Update." In *Vitamins, Nutrition and Cancer,* edited by K. N. Prasad. Basel: Karger, 1984.

Shamberger, R. J., F. F. Baughman, S. L. Kalchert, et al. "Carcinogen-induced Chromosomal Breakage Decreased by Antioxidants." *Proceedings of the National Academy of Sciences* 70 (1973): 1461–1463.

Shklar, G., J. Schwartz, D. Trickler, et al. "Regression of Experimental Cancer by Oral Administration of Combined *d*-α-tocopherol and β-carotene." *Nutrition and Cancer* 12 (1989): 321–325.

Slaga, T. J. "Multistage Skin Carcinogenesis and Specificity of Inhibitors." In *Modulation and Mediation of Cancer by Vitamins,* edited by F. L. Meyskens, Jr., and K. N. Prasad. Basel: Karger, 1983.

Sporn, M. B. "Retinoids and Carcinogenesis." *Nutritional Reviews* 35 (1977): 65–69.

Sporn, M. B., A. B. Roberts, and D. S. Goodman, eds. *The Retinoids.* Orlando, Fla.: Academic Press, 1984.

World Cancer Research Fund. *Nutrition and the Prevention of Cancer: A Global Perspective.* Washington, D.C.: American Institute of Cancer, 1997.

Wu, D., M. Meydani, A. A. Beharka, M. Serafini, K. R. Martin, and S. M. Meydani. "In Vitro Supplementation with Different Tocopherol Homologues Can Affect the Functions of Immune Cells in Old Mice." *Free Radical Biology and Medicine* 28 (2000): 643–651.

About the Authors

Kedar N. Prasad, Ph.D., is a tenured professor in the Department of Radiology at the University of Colorado School of Medicine in Denver. He is also the director of the Center for Vitamins and Cancer Research at the university. He is an eminent scientist who has spent more than thirty years researching cancer and other illnesses and is internationally known for his landmark work in the area of micronutrient supplementation, especially as it relates to cancer and neurodegenerative diseases.

Dr. Prasad received an undergraduate degree in biology and chemistry, a master's degree in zoology, and a doctorate in radiation biology at the University of Iowa in Iowa City. He began his career in basic neurological science at the Brookhaven National Laboratory on Long Island, New York. His major academic interests are in the areas of nutrition and cancer, nutrition and neurodegenerative diseases, genes regulating differentiation in nerve cells, and genes regulating degeneration in neurons.

He has been elected a Fellow of the American College of Nutrition and has been a member of many scientific study sections for the National Institutes of Health and the National Science Foundation. He served as president of the International Association for Vitamin and Nutritional Oncology from 1985 to 1989. Dr. Prasad is also an active member of several professional academic organizations, including the Radiation Research Society, Society for Experimental Biology and Medicine, American Society for Cell Biology, American Association for Cancer Research, International Society of Developmental Neuroscience, American Society for Pharmacology and Experimental Therapeutics, International Brain Research Organization, American Society for Neurochemistry, and the International Society for Nutrition and Cancer. He is president of the latter society.

Dr. Prasad has an extraordinary academic track record, and he manages an active university-based research laboratory funded by the National Institutes of Health. He is a prolific scientific writer and has published more than two hundred articles and more than eighty abstracts. He also has been an editor and/or author of fifteen major books on nutrition and cancer, radiation biology, and neurobiology.

K. Che Prasad, M.S., M.D., received his bachelor's degree with highest honors in human integrative biology from the University of California at Berkeley. He was elected to Phi Beta Kappa as a junior and made an original discovery that α-tocopheryl succinate (vitamin E) enhances the effects of naturally occurring substances, such as adenosine 3',5'-cyclic monophosphate (cAMP), on the growth inhibition and differentiation of melanoma cells. After receiving his undergraduate degree, K. Che Prasad entered the joint medical program administered by the University of California at Berkeley and the University of California at San Francisco, from which he received a master's degree in health and medical sciences and a doctor of medicine.

In 1997 Dr. Prasad began a residency in anatomical and surgical pathology at the University of California, San Francisco, where he has a fellowship in surgical pathology. He is a member of the College of American Pathologists, the American Society of Clinical Pathologists, the United States Academy of Pathology, and the Canadian Academy of Pathology.

Index